UP TO DATE ON TINNITUS

Edited by **Fayez Bahmad Jr**

Up to Date on Tinnitus
Edited by Fayez Bahmad Jr

Published by InTech
Janeza Trdine 9, 51000 Rijeka, Croatia

Publishing Process Manager Romana Vukelic

Technical Editor Teodora Smiljanic

Cover Designer InTech Design Team

Additional hard copies can be obtained from orders@intechopen.com

Up to Date on Tinnitus, Edited by Fayez Bahmad Jr
p. cm.
ISBN 978-953-307-655-3

For EU product safety concerns:
IN TECH d.o.o., Prolaz Marije Krucifikse Kozulić 3, 51000 Rijeka, Croatia,
info@intechopen.com or visit our website at intechopen.com.

Meet the editor

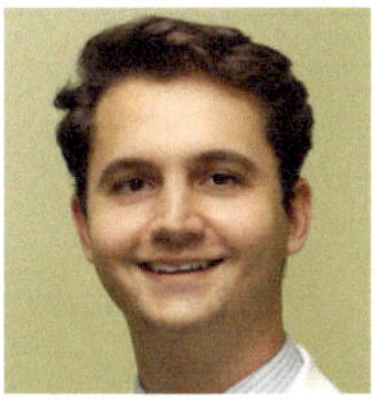

Dr. Fayez Bahmad is Editor In Chief of the traditional The International Tinnitus Journal. He went through the ENT Residency Program at University of Brasilia Hospital (Otolaryngology) and received his PhD at University of Brasilia Medical School under the orientation of Professor Carlos A. Oliveira, MD, PhD. He was awarded the prestigious Schuknecht Prize at the International Otopathology Society Meeting held in Boston in 2003. He was a Fellow in Otology & Neurotology at Massachusetts Eye & Ear Infirmary, and Fellow in Human Genetics at Seidman Laboratory, Department of Genetics, both at Harvard Medical School when he was engaged in projects under the mentorship of Professor Saumil N. Merchant MD, PhD, one of the foremost professors and researchers in otology and otopathology. Professor Oliveira is well known for establishing otopathology laboratory in his department, and for having one of the most successful researcher groups in Otology in Brazil and South America.

Contents

Preface

Up to Date on Tinnitus is directed toward the clinicians and provides detailed information on diagnosis of many different forms of tinnitus and their treatment as well as an overview of what is known about their pathophysiology.

Accordingly, this book does not cover all the different theories and management of tinnitus, but it does present an up-to-date information for those who deal with tinnitus in their clinical praxis such as otolaryngologists, neurologists, psychiatrists, neurosurgeons, clinical audiologists, dentists, and psychologists.

This book encompasses both theoretical background of the different forms of tinnitus and detailed knowledge on state-of-the-art treatment of tinnitus, written for clinicians by clinicians and researchers. Realizing the complexity of tinnitus has highlighted the importance of interdisciplinary research. Therefore, each of the authors contributing to the "Up-to-date on Tinnitus" were chosen from many specialties of medicine, like surgery, psychology, and neuroscience, and came from diverse areas of expertise, such as Neurology, Neurosurgery, Audiology, Otolaryngology, Psychiatry, Clinical and Experimental Psychology, Pharmacology, Dentistry, and Neuroscience.

Many structures of the body, such as the ear, the auditory nervous system, the somatosensory system, other parts of the brain, muscles of the head and the neck are directly or indirectly involved in different forms of tinnitus. Treating and understanding the pathology of tinnitus requires better knowledge of otopathology and the involvement of many specialties of medicine, such as surgery, psychology, and neuroscience. Hearing loss may occur by genetic defects, presbycusis, viral or bacterial infection, temporal bone trauma, noise exposure, administration of ototoxical agents, but the cause of subjective tinnitus is often unknown. Severe tinnitus is often accompanied by symptoms, such as hyperacusis (lowered tolerance to sound) and distortion of sounds. Affective disorders such as phonophobia (fear of sound) and depression often occur in individuals with severe tinnitus. With such differences in symptoms, it is unreasonable to expect that a single cause can be responsible for severe tinnitus, which is yet another factor that makes managing the tinnitus patient a challenge for health care professionals.

Chapter 1 provides the reader with current knowledge on tinnitus and hearing loss; Chapters 2 and 3 describe the relation between stomatognathic system and the development of tinnitus and provide details on how tinnitus can appear in patients suffering with temporo mandibular disorders; Chapter 4 discusses the outcome of somatic tinnitus in clinical practice, an ideal integrated management.

Chapter 5 introduces possibilities for tinnitus management in the emergency department; Chapter 6 presents a critical overview of the Medico-Legal Decision Making in NIHL-Related Tinnitus; Chapter 7 discusses the components of Metabolic Syndrome and Their Relation with Tinnitus; Chapters 8 and 9 offer new alternative treatments of tinnitus as home medical device for Tinnitus Treatment and Bhramari Pranayama as Alternative Treatments; Finally, Chapter 10 presents the "Emotional Side" of Subjective Tinnitus.

It is a huge challenge to translate the results from basic research into clinical practice and all the authors have attempted to present the pathophysiological model in a clear way. Still the principles on which it is based and its mechanisms are complex and their understanding requires knowledge from various areas of neuroscience and the fact that tinnitus is not a simple disease but a group of diseases means tinnitus cannot be effectively treated by a single approach, and several disciplines of health care must be involved.

The Editor would like to thank Ms Romana Vukelic for her support in the preparation of this book.

Special thanks are due to Professor Carlos Oliveira for making valuable discussions and suggestions during the editing of the book.

Fayez Bahmad Jr, MD, PhD
Health Science Faculty,
University of Brasilia,
Brazil

Part 1

Tinnitus and Hearing Loss

1

Tinnitus and Hearing Loss

Fayez Bahmad Jr, Carlos Augusto C.P. Oliveira and Lisiane Holdefer
University of Brasilia Medical School,
Brasilia -Distrito Federal,
Brasil

1. Introduction

Tinnitus is a symptom present in approximately 15% of the world, and this proportion increases to 33% in individuals over 60 years Jastreboff and Hanzel, 1993). It carries a negative impact on quality of life for 20% of them.

May be associated with more than 300 diseases (Ganança et al, 1994), with a hearing loss of the most common (Hiller and Goebel, 2006). Only 80-10% of patients with tinnitus have normal hearing (Barnea et al, 1990), while 85 to 96% have some degree of hearing loss (Fowler, 1994; Sanchez e Ferrari, 2002).

The influence of hearing loss in the degree of suffering of tinnitus remains no consensus (Baskell and Coles, 1999). Findings relate tinnitus severity to hearing loss at high frequencies (Weisz et al, 2004). Mazurek et al (2010) found a significant correlation between the degree of hearing loss and tinnitus loudness. They found that patients with decompensated chronic tinnitus had more hearing loss than those with compensated tinnitus. The study concluded had evidence that indirectly support the hypothesis that the degree of hearing loss affects the severity of tinnitus (Mazurek et al, 2010).

Clinically significant hearing loss in patients with tinnitus was associated with anxiety and depression as a reaction to hearing loss that could interfere with the impact of tinnitus (McKinney et al, 1999). However it is not possible to say whether the hearing loss is only one cause of tinnitus or whether it also influences the severity and handicap (Davis, 1996).

Searches related to gender discomfort is inconclusive. While Davis (1983) observed higher scores for discomfort due to tinnitus in women compared with men (Davis and Cole, 1983 and Coelho et al, 2004), and Hiller and Goebel (2006) a higher intensity and severity of tinnitus annoyance in older men. Méric et al (1998) and Pinto et al (2010) assessed the impact of tinnitus on quality of life and found no correlation between age, sex or duration of tinnitus and the annoyance it causes.

The subjectivity of tinnitus, its symptoms, the different characteristics of each patient and the many causes of tinnitus are issues that require investigation. It is known that hearing loss is one of the largest generators of tinnitus and its pathology and diagnostics must be studied and known to offer the patient the 'most successful treatment option in symptom remission.

It is well established that after lesions of the peripheral auditory receptor, the cochlea, increased spontaneous activity (hyperactivity) develops in central auditory nuclei. This plasticity has been demonstrated in a wide range of animal models, using either mechanically, acoustically, or drug-induced cochlear lesions (Brozoski et al., 2007; Bauer et al., 2008; Dong et al., 2009; Mulders and Robertson, 2009). Hyperactivity has been suggested to be involved in the generation of tinnitus, an auditory phantom perception (Brozoski et al., 2002; Bauer et al., 2008). This hypothesis is supported by the fact that the hyperactivity seems restricted to tonotopic regions broadly corresponding to the area of hearing loss as shown in cochlear nucleus, the central nucleus of the inferior colliculus, and the auditory cortex (Dong et al., 2009; Mulders et al., 2009) and the observation in human studies that there is a strong correlation between the tinnitus pitch and the hearing loss frequencies (Norena et al., 2002; Eggermont and Roberts, 2004).

The study of Mulders et al (2010) indicate a strong effect of stimulation of the medial olivocochlear (OC) system on hyperactivity caused by acoustic trauma. This demonstration that an intrinsic control system can modify maladaptive plastic phenomena in the auditory pathway, could have important clinical implications. If spontaneous hyperactivity is indeed involved in the generation of tinnitus (Brozoski et al., 2002; Bauer et al., 2008), then our results could indicate a beneficial effect of OC system activation on tinnitus. Mulders et al (2010) find that the suppressive effects on spontaneous activity lasted after the stimulation had ceased, is consistent with a role for the OC system in residual inhibition, a temporary reduction of tinnitus experienced in tinnitus patients that persists for a few seconds after masking sounds are turned off (Vernon and Meikle, 2003; Roberts et al., 2008). Likewise, activation of the OC system could be a contributory mechanism to the often beneficial effects of masking sounds on the perception of tinnitus (Jastreboff, 2007; Lugli et al., 2009, Holdefer et al, 2010), since the OC system itself can be activated by sound (Thompson and Thompson, 1991; Lugli et al., 2009).

2. Tinnitus loudness in hearing loss patients

The loudness of tinnitus can be estimated by asking the individual to adjust an external sound so as to match the loudness of the tinnitus. One method is for the listener to first select a sound that is similar to their tinnitus. For example, if the tinnitus is tonal, the listener might adjust the frequency of a pure tone until it matches the pitch of their tinnitus. Then, the external tone is adjusted in level so as to match the loudness of the tinnitus.

Often, the matching sound is presented to the ear opposite to that for which the tinnitus is reported to be louder, so as to avoid the matching sound masking the tinnitus or reducing its loudness. A common finding of such studies is that the tinnitus is matched by a sound with a low sensation level (SL; the level of a sound relative to an individual's absolute threshold), as first described by Fowler in 1941. Fowler reported that most matches were at 5 or 10 dB SL, leading him to describe "the illusion of loudness of tinnitus." Graham and Newby in 1962 found that the majority of people with troublesome tinnitus matched to a level of 5 dB SL or less. Reed in 1960 reported that 41% of tinnitus patients matched to a level of 5 dB SL or less, 69% to a level of 10 dB SL or less, and 87% to a level of 20 dB SL or less. Vernon in 1976 reported no matches higher than 20 dB SL. For a review of other studies showing similar results, see Tyler and Conrad-Armes in 1983. Recently, automated methods for computerized assessment of tinnitus loudness have been described: unsurprisingly, these produced similar results.

These findings led to the idea that tinnitus is usually perceived as soft, rather than as loud, despite causing marked distress for some people. Vernon considered 3 possible explanations for this apparent paradox: first, the method for estimating the loudness of tinnitus may not be valid; second, distress may not be related to loudness; and third, the loudness of the tinnitus may actually be quite high even when the matching sound has a low SL because of the existence of loudness recruitment at the frequency of the matching sound. Loudness recruitment is a phenomenon usually associated with cochlear hearing loss.

For a frequency where a person has a hearing loss, the loudness of a tone or other sound increases more rapidly than normal once the sound level is increased above the absolute threshold, and at high levels, the loudness is similar to what would be experienced by a person with normal hearing. Thus, if the listener has a hearing loss at the frequency of the tone used to obtain a tinnitus match, the loudness of the matching tone may be moderately high, although its SL is low.

The explanation in terms of loudness recruitment was explored further by Goodwin and Johnson in 1980. They tested 9 adults with tonal tinnitus, all of whom had a "normal" audiometric threshold (20 dB HL or better, where hearing level [HL] is the level of a sound relative to the absolute threshold of humans with "normal" hearing at that frequency) for at least 1 frequency. They compared loudness matches to the tinnitus using 2 methods: 1) the frequency of the matching tone was chosen to match the pitch of the tinnitus. This was called the matching frequency. For all listeners, the hearing loss was 25 dB or more at this frequency. The matching tone was presented to the ear opposite to the ear in which the tinnitus was loudest. This was called the traditional method. 2) The frequency of the matching tone was chosen as the closest audiometric frequency to the matching frequency for which the absolute threshold was 20 dB HL or better. This was called the normal frequency. It was assumed that loudness recruitment would be small or absent at the normal frequency. In this case, the matching tone was presented to the same ear as the ear in which the tinnitus was loudest because it was assumed that the matching tone would have a negligible effect in masking the tinnitus or reducing its loudness. This was called the proposed method.

For every listener, the matching SLs were higher for the proposed method than for the traditional method. For the traditional method, the matches ranged from 1 to 20 dB SL, with a mean of 6.6 dB SL. For the proposed method, the matches ranged from 8 to 50 dB SL, with a mean of 33.4 dB SL. Goodwin and Johnson concluded that loudness recruitment did have a clear influence on the tinnitus matches and that the proposed method gave more realistic estimates of the loudness of the tinnitus. Their results suggested that tinnitus is usually soft to medium in loudness.

A similar study was conducted by Tyler and Conrad-Armes, who additionally used formulae based on abnormal loudness functions and uncomfortable loudness levels to calculate the loudness of their matches in sones. However, the values obtained depended strongly on the formula used; the mean calculated loudness of the tinnitus ranged from 6 (a low-to-moderate loudness) to 76 sones (rather loud).

It is well known that, for many tinnitus patients, the loudness of tinnitus can be reduced by external sounds. If the external sound is sufficiently intense, the tinnitus may be rendered inaudible, that is, it may be masked. Indeed, reduction of loudness or masking of tinnitus forms part of many methods for alleviating the effects of tinnitus. However, there have been few quantitative studies of the influence of background sounds on the loudness of tinnitus. Furthermore, it seems that this effect is variable between individuals.

3. Tinnitus and noise loud exposure

Hearing loss and tinnitus are the two most prevalent service-connected disabilities for U.S. veterans, including those who served in Operation Iraqi Freedom or Operation Enduring

Freedom (Folmer et al, 2011). Currently, in the Department of Veterans Affairs (VA), more than 570,000 veterans are service-connected for hearing loss and more than 639,000 are service-connected for tinnitus, which means they qualify for monthly compensation and/or VA clinical services related to these auditory disorders.

Because many veterans were exposed to loud sounds during military service, the author anticipated that they would exhibit higher (that is, poorer) pure tone thresholds than age-matched groups of nonveterans and predicted that males with histories of loud noise exposure would exhibit higher pure tone thresholds than age-matched males who reported less noise exposure. Finally, they hypothesized that the chronic tinnitus prevalence would be significantly greater among male veterans than the prevalence among male nonveterans and that tinnitus prevalence among males with histories of loud noise exposure would be greater than that among age-matched males with less noise exposure.

Tinnitus is the perception of ringing, buzzing, hissing, or other noises in the ears or head in the absence of external sources for these sounds. These perceptions can be transient, intermittent, occasional, or constant. "Chronic" tinnitus is present all or most of the time during a person's waking hours. Like sensorineural hearing loss, chronic tinnitus more likely occurs in middle-aged and older people, especially those who have been repeatedly exposed to loud sounds without using hearing protection devices.

Analysis of data from Folmer et al in 2011, showed that the overall chronic tinnitus prevalence is greater for veterans (11.7%) than the prevalence for nonveterans (5.4%), with statistically significant differences in the 50 to 59 and 60 to 69 age groups. Also, the prevalence of tinnitus among males who reported a noise exposure history is significantly higher than the prevalence among males who reported less noise exposure. However, with few exceptions, the pure tone hearing thresholds for veterans did not differ significantly from nonveteran audiograms; males who reported more noise exposure did not have substantially worse hearing than males the same age with less noise exposure.

These surprising audiometric results probably occurred because the larger effect of age in our decade-by-decade comparisons obscured the small differences in pure tone thresholds, if they exist between groups (veterans vs nonveterans or noise-exposed vs non-noise-exposed males).

In the near future, hearing loss and tinnitus will likely remain the most prevalent service-connected disabilities among all U.S. veterans. In addition, increasing numbers of veterans will probably seek and receive VA compensation and medical and rehabilitative services for these conditions. As they plan for future costs of healthcare and compensation, the Veterans Health Administration (VHA) and the VBA should be able to use results of this study and its estimates of audiometric thresholds and tinnitus prevalence among male veterans in the United States.

4. Tinnitus after resection of Vestibular Schwannoma (VS)

Slater et al in 1987 reported that 28% of respondents (n = 255) to a questionnaire survey about tinnitus agreed that external sound could result in tinnitus being more "noticeable." In particular, we have noted clinically that the subgroup of individuals who have undergone surgical resection of VS report that their tinnitus is much more troublesome in noisy environments.

For these patients, a noise presented to the "dead" ear would not be heard, so it is unlikely that the noise would have any influence on the tinnitus. However, a noise presented to the functioning ear might influence the loudness of tinnitus, although it would be unable to mask it at the cochlear level. To our knowledge, this possibility has not been systematically investigated.

Cope et al in 2011 showed that, for listeners who are unilaterally deaf after surgery for VS, the loudness of the tinnitus heard in the deaf ear usually increases with increasing level of a noise applied to the "good" ear. The threshold-equalizing-noise (TEN) started to lead to an increase in the loudness of the tinnitus when presented at a level approximately 15 dB below the matching level in quiet, after which higher levels of the TEN produced progressive increases in loudness. The authors showed relatively consistent effect across participants (with one exception) suggesting a common underlying cause.

There were at least 2 plausible and not mutually exclusive explanations for the effect of background noise on tinnitus loudness for VS participants. The first is that it reflects a plausible perceptual interpretation of the sensory evidence. All perception may be regarded as hypothesis driven, with the brain attempting to arrive at the best possible interpretation of the sensory evidence.

For a target sound (an acoustic sound as opposed to the perception of tinnitus) to be audible in the presence of a broadband background sound, the level of the target must be comparable to the level of the background at the output of at least one auditory filter.

Returning to tinnitus, if tinnitus remains audible in the presence of increasing levels of background sound, as it did for our listeners with VS, then the most plausible perceptual interpretation is that the source of the tinnitus is increasing in intensity with increasing background level, and this may give rise to the perception of increasing loudness of the tinnitus. Note that the perceptual processes involved do not involve conscious reasoning, rather they reflect "unconscious inference"

The action of the efferent pathways in the auditory system, especially the medial olivo-cochlear (MOC) system. One role of the MOC system is to regulate the gain provided by the active mechanism in the cochlea, by controlling the operation of the outer hair cells. With increasing input sound level, signals from the MOC system cause a reduction of the gain of the active mechanism, effectively acting as a form of automatic gain control, provided that the auditory system is functioning normally.

The regulatory signals from the MOC system are taken into account in interpreting the information flowing from the auditory nerve to higher centers, thus allowing the brain to arrive at an accurate and consistent interpretation of the magnitudes of sounds.

For the listeners with VS, MOC signals would still have been sent from the brainstem, but they would not have reached the cochlea because the efferent system was severed at the VIIIth nerve level as part of the surgery (and even if the cochlea did respond, this would be no resulting signal at higher levels in the auditory system because the auditory nerve itself was severed). The signals from the higher centers would have carried "instructions" to decrease the gain of the active mechanism as the level of the noise in the "good" ear was increased. However, the abnormal activity in the auditory pathway that gave rise to the tinnitus was presumably not affected by the signals from the MOC system. The unchanging tinnitus signal, in combination with MOC "instructions" to decrease the gain, may have resulted in the increasing loudness of the tinnitus with increasing background level.

This finding that the loudness of tinnitus increases with increasing background noise level in the contralateral ear of participants with VS has important clinical implications. Patients who are about to receive treatment for VS, or have recently received treatment for VS, should be counseled about this at an appropriate point in their treatment pathway, and this counseling should raise the possibility that the increase in the loudness of tinnitus may affect their ability to concentrate on speech in noise.

Also, some clinicians faced with a VS patient with severe tinnitus may consider the use of wideband therapy in the contralateral ear: suggest that this intervention may well be unhelpful and doomed to failure, and indeed, some protocols (specifically tinnitus retraining therapy) already indicate that this is contraindicated. It should be noted that individuals who had undergone surgical resection and were rendered unilaterally deaf after treatment; it is not known whether those treated with hearing preservation surgery or radiologic techniques have the same experience.

5. Tinnitus in otosclerosis patients

Many papers have been written about tinnitus outcome after stapes surgery. However, none has attempted to quantify the intensity of the symptom pre- and postoperatively in order to evaluate the influence of surgery on the degree of annoyance caused by tinnitus. Severe disabling tinnitus (SDT) is defined by Shulman as a symptom severe enough to disrupt the patient´s routine and to pre-vent him from performing his daily tasks.

In 1953, Heller and Bergman (9) showed that over 90% of normal-hearing people reported tinnitus when placed in a soundproof cabin. However, the symptom did not cause any discomfort to those patients in daily life. Being so, it becomes necessary to separate commom garden variety tinnitus from serious, disrupting ones.

Shulman (10) coined the term severe disabling tinnitus (SDT) for a symptom that is severe enough to disrupt the patient´s routine and to keep him from performing his daily tasks. Usually, this kind of patient seeks medical attention because of his tinnitus, while in less severe cases the symptom is mentioned during medical consultation for other problems.

Tinnitus is certainly very common among otosclerosis patients; some of them report very intense annoyance from the symptom and ask what will happen to the symptom after stapes surgery.

We tried to quantify the intensity of tinnitus in otosclerosis patients pre- and postoperatively by means of a visual analogue scale (VAS) going from 1 (very low intensity) to 10 (unbearable intensity). We considered SDT as having an intensity of 7-10 on the VAS. By comparing the tinnitus score before and after stapes surgery for otosclerosis, we tried to determine the influence of the surgical procedure on SDT. The results of this study are reported below.

We applied a VAS, in which 1 meant a very low intensity and 10 an unbearable intensity for the symptom of tinnitus, to 48 consecutive otosclerosis patients before and after stapes surgery. We considered SDT as yielding a score of 7 or above on the VAS.

In all patients pure-tone audiometry and a word discrimination test were performed pre- and postoperatively.

Forty-four patients underwent stapedotomy and 4 stapedectomy. Hearing results were evaluated by comparing the pre- and postoperative four-tone average air-bone gaps. The influence of surgery on SDT was measured by comparing pre- and postoperative scores for the symptom on the VAS. The operative notes were carefully reviewed for any problem occuring during surgery.

The VAS was applied 4-10 months after surgery. We considered significant a score improvement of $\geq$2 points on the VAS.Twenty-five patients were contacted 14-48 months after surgery and were asked about the tinnitus status at this late follow-up time.

The protocol was approved by the ethics committee on research involving human subjects of our institution.

6. Results

There were 29 female and 19 male patients. Forty-four of the 48 patients reported tinnitus preoperatively (91.6%). Mean age was 44.5 years (range 16-62).
SDT was present in 19 patients preoperatively (39.6%) and female patients tended to report more SDT than male counterparts (55.5% of female and 15.8% of male patients).

Patients with SDT	19
Total remission	10 (52.6%)
Significant improvement	6 (31.7%)
Slight improvement	1 (5.2%)
No change	2 (10.4%)

Table 1. SDT: postoperative outcome

Preoprative air-bone gap in patients with SDT	n	Total remission
>30 dB	14	8 (57.14%)
<30 dB	5	2 (40.0%)

Table 2. Preoperative air-bone gap and postoperative SDT remission

Air-bone gap	n	Total remission	Significant improvement	Slight improvement	No improvement
0-20 dB	17 (89.46%)	9 (52.9%)	7 (41.2%)	0	1 (5.84%)
>20 dB	2 (10.52%)	0	0	1 (50%)	1 (50%)

Table 3. Postoperative air-bone gap and SDT

Overall 40 (90.9%) tinnitus patients reported postoperative improvement and 4 (9.09%) noted no change in tinnitus. None said the symptom was worse.
Table 1 shows postoperative tinnitus outcome of the 19 SDT patients. Ten of the 19 tinnitus patients reported total remission of tinnitus after surgery and 6 had a significant improvement (at least 2 points on the VAS). One reported a slight improvement and 2 noted no change in the symptom.
The intensity of preoperative tinnitus was not related to the preoperative air-bone gap (mean air-bone gap of 34.3 dB for SDT and 31.4 dB for less intense tinnitus). However, larger preoperative air-bone gaps seemed to predict better postoperative improvement in SDT (table 2) when a good hearing result was achieved. Smaller postoperative air-bone gaps correlated with more remission and improvement of SDT postoperatively (table3).
There was a trend for lower preoperative bone conduction levels to correlate with preoperative SDT (44.1% of patients with a four-tone average bone conduction level below 40 dB had preoperative SDT while 28.5% of patients with a preoperative four-tone average bone conduction level above 40 dB had SDT).
Twenty-five patients (7 SDT) contacted 14-48 months after surgery said their tinnitus status had not changed since surgery.
There were no untoward events during surgery and no postoperative complications other than 6 patients with an air-bone gap above 20 dB were seen.

7. Comments

In 1999, Oliveira ET AL (11) applied a tinnitus questionnaire that included a VAS to all new patients seen at the Otology Clinic of the Brasília University Hospital for a 6-month period of time. Five hundred tinnitus patients were identified. These patients had presbycusis, chronic otitis media, otosclerosis, acoustic trauma, Menière´s disease, ototoxicity and vestibular schwannoma in this order of frequency. However, 81% of the tinnitus patients had a very mild symptom and only mentioned tinnitus because they were asked about it. Eighteen percent had a mild symptom they could tolerate well or were easily relieved with routine medical treatment. Only 1% had tinnitus that was very intense (above 7 on the VAS), dirupting the patient´s routine, and they were refractory to medical treatment (central vasodilators, vestibular suppressants, calcium channel blockers, anticholinergics, anticonvulsants). To sum up, tinnitus is a very common symptom among patients of an otology clinic but only 1% of these patients have SDT.

Otosclerosis was the 3rd most frequent diagnosis listed above and we have found an incidence of tinnitus (91.6%) in our 48 otosclerosis patients similar to the one in the general population (9). However, 39.6% of our otosclerosis patients had SDT as compared to 1% in the patients of our otology clinic. Therefore, otosclerosis seems to be strongly associated with SDT.

Otosclerosis patients who have SDT are the ones who always ask the doctor what will happen to their tinnitus after stapes surgery and often mention tinnitus relief as their priority. Because all papers published up to now (1-8) had not targeted SDT, we undertook the present study.

Our results allow the following statements:

1. Otosclerosis is a major cause for SDT. How the otosclerosis process leads to severe tinnitus remains to be clarified.
2. Stapes surgery (namely stapedotomy, because 44 of our 48 patients had this operation performed) can totally relieve SDT in roughly 50% of cases and significantly improve another 31%. About 10.4% of SDT patients will not have any relief after stapes surgery. These patients probably have already developed a paradoxical memory in the medial temporal lobe system as proposed by Shulman ET AL (10) and will not respond to any treatment of the peripheral organ.
3. Because larger air-bone gaps preoperatively predict better tinnitus improvement when the stapes surgery results in smaller postoperative air-bone gaps (tables 2 and 3), we suggest that the masking effect produced by better postoperative hearing is probably responsible for the tinnitus improvement.
4. Since 25 tinnitus patients (7 SDT) contacted up to 48 months after surgery said their tinnitus status had not changed compared to the early follow-up situation, it is safe to say that the influence of stapes surgery on SDT in otosclerosis patients is long-lasting.
5. Worsening of SDT after stapes surgery is unlikely provided an atraumatic procedure was performed.

8. References

[1] Jastreboff PJ, Hazell JWP. A neurophysiological approach to tinnitus clinical implications. Br J Audiol. 1993. 27 (1): 7-17.

[2] Ganança MM, Caovilla H, Fukuda Y, Munhoz MSL. Afecções e Síndromes Otoneurológicas. In: Lopes Filho, O. & Campos, C. A. H. Tratado de Otorrinolaringologia. São Paulo, Roca, 1994, 835-843.

[3] Hiller W, Goebel G. Factors Influencing Tinnitus Loudness and Annoyance. Arch Otolaryngol Head and Neck Surg, 2006. 132: 1323-30. 1323-30.

[4] Barnea G, Attias J, Gold S, Shahar A. Tinnitus with normal hearing sensitivity: extended high-frequency audiometry and auditory nerv brain-sterm-evoked responses. Audiology, 1990. 29: 36-45.

[5] Fowler EP. Head noises in normal and disordered ears: significance, measurement, differentiation and treatment. Arch Otoryngol, 1994. 39: 498

[6] Sanchez TG, Ferrari GMS. O controle do zumbido por meio de prótese auditiva: sugestões para otimização do uso. Pró-Fono Revista de Atualização Científica, 2002. 14(1): 111-8.

[7] Baskill JL, Coles RRA. Relationship between tinnitus loudness and severity. In: Hazell J. (ed.) Proceedings Sixth International Tinnitus Seminar. Cambridge, UK: The Tinnitus and Hyperacusis Centre, 1999. 424-8.

[8] Weisz N, Voss S, Berg P, Elbert T. Abnormal auditory mismatch response in tinnitus sufferes with high-frequency hearing loss is associated with subjective distress level. BMC Neurosci. 2004. 5:8-16.

[9] Mazurek B, Olze H, Haupt H, Szezepek AJ. The more the worse: the grade of noise-induced hearing loss associates with the severity of tinnitus. Int J Environ. Res Pub Helth. 2010. 7:3071-9.

[10] McKinney, CJ, Hazell JWP, Graham RL. An evaluation of the TRT method. . In: Hazell, J. (ed.) Proceedings Sixth International Tinnitus Seminar. Cambridge, UK: The Tinnitus and Hyperacusis Centre, 1999. 9-105.

[11] Davis A. The etiology of tinnitus: risk factors for tinnitus in the UK population- a possible role for conductive pathologies. In: Reich, G. E. e Vernon, J. A. P (ed.) Proceedings Fifth International Tinnitus Seminars, 1996. 38-45.

[12] Davis A. Hearing disorders in the population: first phase findings of the MRC national study of hearing. In: Hearing Science and Hearing Disorders. Lutman, M. E; Haggard, M. P. Churchill Livingstone: 1983. 35-60.

[13] Coelho CCB, Sanchez TG, Bento RF. Características do zumbido em pacientes atendidos em um serviço de referência. Arq Int Otorrinolaringol. 2004. (3): 284-92.

[14] Méric C, Gatner M, Collet l, Chéry-Croze S. Psychopathological profile of tinnitus sufferers: evidence concerning the relationship between tinnitus features and impact on life. Audiol Neurootol. 1998. 3(4): 240-52.

[15] Pinto PCL, Sanchez TG, Tomita S. The impact of gender, age and hearing loss on tinnitus severity. Braz J Otorhinolayng. 2010. 76(1): 18-24.

[16] Bauer CA, Turner JG, Caspary DM, Myers KS, Brozoski TJ. Tinnitus and inferior colliculus activity in chinchillas related to three distinct patterns of cochlear trauma. J Neurosci Res, 2008. 86:2564 –2578.

[17] Brozoski TJ, Bauer CA, Caspary DM. Elevated fusiform cell activity in the dorsal cochlear nucleus of chinchillas with psychophysical evidence of tinnitus. J Neurosci, 2002. 22:2383–2390.

[18] Brozoski TJ, Ciobanu L, BauerCA Central neural activity in rats with tinnitus evaluated with manganese-enhanced magnetic resonance imaging (MEMRI). Hear Res, 2007. 228:168 –179.

[19] Dong S, Mulders WH, Rodger J, Robertson D. Changes in neuronal activity and gene expression in guinea-pig auditory brainstem after unilateral partial hearing loss. Neuroscience, 2009. 159:1164 –1174.

[20] Eggermont JJ, Roberts LE. The neuroscience of tinnitus. Trends Neurosci, 2004. 27: 676 – 682.

[21] Mulders WH, Paolini AG, Needham K, Robertson D. Synaptic responses in cochlear nucleus neurons evoked by activation of the olivocochlear system. Hear Res, 2009. 256:85–92.
[22] Mulders WH, Robertson D. Hyperactivity in the auditory midbrain after acoustic trauma: dependence on cochlear activity. Neuroscience, 2009. 164:733–746.
[23] Norena A, Micheyl C, Che´ry-Croze S, Collet L. Psychoacoustic characterization of the tinnitus spectrum: implications for the underlying mechanisms of tinnitus. Audiol Neurootol, 2002. 7:358 –369.
[24] Mulders WHAM, Seluakumaran K, Roberson S. Efferent Modulation of Hyperactivity in Inferior ColliculusJ. Neurosci., July 14, 2010. 30(28):9578 –9587.
[25] Thompson AM, Thompson GC. Posteroventral cochlear nucleus projections to olivocochlear neurons. J Comp Neurol, 1991. 303:267–285.
[26] Jastreboff MM. Sound therapies for tinnitus management. Prog Brain Res, 2007. 166:435–440.
[27] Lugli M, Romani R, Ponzi S, Bacciu S, Parmigiani S. The windowed sound therapy: a new empirical approach for an effectiv personalized treatment of tinnitus. Int Tinnitus J, 2009. 15:51- 61.
[28] Vernon JA, Meikle MB. Tinnitus: clinical measurement. Otolaryngol Clin North Am, 2003. 36:293–305.
[29] Roberts LE, Moffat G, Baumann M, Ward LM, Bosnyak DJ. Residual inhibition functions overlap tinnitus spectra and the region of auditory threshold shift. J Assoc Res Otolaryngol, 2008. 9:417- 435.
[30] Holdefer L, Oliveira CACP, Venosa AR. Sucesso no tratamento do zumbido em grupo. Rev Bras Otorrino, 2010. 76(1):102-6.
[31] Folmer RL, McMillan GP, Austin DF, Henry JA. Audiometric thresholds and prevalence of tinnitus among male veterans in the United States: Data from the National Health and Nutrition Examination Survey, 1999-2006. J Rehabil Res Dev. 2011;48(5):503-16.
[32] Cope TE, Baguley DM, Moore BC. Tinnitus loudness in quiet and noise after resection of vestibular schwannoma. Otol Neurotol. 2011 Apr;32(3):488-96.
[33] Fowler EP. Tinnitus aurium in the light of recent research. Ann Otol Rhinol Laryngol 1941;50:139-58.
[34] Graham JT, Newby HA. Acoustical characteristics of tinnitus. An analysis. Arch Otolaryngol 1962;75:162-7.
[35] Reed GF. An audiometric study of two hundred cases of subjective tinnitus. Arch Otolaryngol 1960;71:84-94.
[36] Vernon J. The loudness (?) of tinnitus. Hear Speech Act 1976;44:17-9.
[37] Tyler RS, Conrad-Armes D. The determination of tinnitus loudness considering the effects of recruitment. J Speech Hear Res 1983;26:59-72.
[38] Henry JA, Rheinsburg B, Owens KK, Ellingson RM. New instrumentation for automated tinnitus psychoacoustic assessment. Acta Otolaryngol 2006;556:34-8.
[39] Fowler EP. A method for the early detection of otosclerosis. Arch Otolaryngol 1936;24:731-41.
[40] Steinberg JC, Gardner MB. The dependency of hearing impairment on sound intensity. J Acoust Soc Am 1937;9:11-23.
[41] Goodwin PE, Johnson RM. The loudness of tinnitus. Acta Otolaryngol 1980;90:353-59.
[42] Slater R, Terry M, Davis B. Tinnitus: A Guide for Sufferers and Professionals. Beckenham, UK: Croon Helm, 1987.

Part 2

Tinnitus and Stomatognathic System

2

Tinnitus and Temporomandibular Disorders

Kengo Torii
Nippon Dental University
Japan

1. Introduction

Temporomandibular disorders (TMDs) are a group of related disorders of the masticatory system (the masticatory musculature and the temporomandibular joint). The most frequent symptom is pain, usually localized in the muscles of mastication, the preauricular region, and the temporomandibular joint (TMJ). Patients often complain of jaw ache, earache, headache, and facial pain. In addition to pain, patients with these disorders frequently have limited or asymmetric jaw movement and joint sounds that are described as clicking or crepitus (McNeill, 1990). The causes of TMDs remain unclear, and numerous factors have been implicated.

The first description of the relationship between TMJ dysfunction and aural symptoms is thought to have been made by Costen in 1934. Costen reported various clinical cases of patients with ear and nasal symptoms; he summarized his findings by stating that hearing tests showed a mild type of catarrhal otitis with eustachian tube involvement (usually simple obstruction). The prognosis of such cases reportedly depended on these factors: (a) the accuracy with which refitted dentures relieved the abnormal pressure on the joint; and (b) the extent of the injury to the tube and to the condyle, meniscus, and joint capsule. A more general acknowledgement of the relationship between ear symptoms and TMJ dysfunction was subsequently made (Costen, 1934, 1936, 1944). Sicher reported that from an anatomical perspective, the eustachian tube cannot be compressed during the closure of the mandible; neither can the opening action of the tensor palati muscle on the tube be impaired in this condition, making Costen's theory impossible (Sicher, 1948). Schwartz theorized that contractive muscle spasms may cause pain as a direct result of myofascial trigger mechanisms and by referred routes (Schwartz, 1956).

2. Tinnitus and treatment for TMDs

After Schwarzt's proposal, Dolowitz et al. reported that muscle exercises were effective for the relief of aural symptoms, especially ear fullness (44 out of 47 diagnosed patients) and tinnitus (40 out of 43 diagnosed patients). Various therapies have since been tried for the relief of TMD symptoms, including aural symptoms (Dolowitz et al., 1964). These therapies include selective grinding of the teeth, bite plate, biofeedback training, thermotherapy and muscle training (Koskinnen et al., 1980; Principato & Barwell, 1978). Parker and Chole reported that tinnitus and vertigo were significantly more prevalent among a TMD group than among either of their control groups (Parker & Chole, 1995). Erlandsson et al. reported that stomatognathic treatment (occlusal splint, occlusal adjustment, and exercise therapy) and biofeedback treatment seemed to have some positive effects in a subgroup of tinnitus patients (with normal hearing) (Erlandsson et al., 1991). Rubinstein performed extensive studies of TMD and tinnitus and made the following conclusions: (1) 46 % of the patients who had received stomatognathic treatment reported no tinnitus or reduced tinnitus a few months after treatment. A two-year follow-up showed that the improvement persisted in most of those who had benefited from the treatment. (2) Frequent headaches, fatigue/tenderness in the jaw muscles, clinical findings of pain upon palpation of the masticatory muscles, impaired mandibular mobility, and signs of parafunctions were more prevalent among tinnitus patients than among an epidemiological sampling. (3) The awareness of diurnal bruxism and a feeling of jaw tenderness/fatigue may be related to fluctuating tinnitus, vertigo and hyperacusis. (4) The evaluation of treatment outcome showed some improvements at the group level: a decrease in tinnitus, mood improvement, and a reduction in clinical signs of the dysfunction of the masticatory system. And (5), a strong relationship existed between tinnitus complaints and several symptoms of TMD. In summary, a relatively low severity of tinnitus, normal hearing, and fluctuations in the tinnitus intensity were good predictors of the psychological, stomatognathic, and cervical treatment outcome (Rubinstein, 1993). Wright and Bifano reported that 38 % of their clinic's patients reported coexisting tinnitus; among the 93 subjects included in their study, 56 % reported that their tinnitus resolved after TMD treatment, 30 % reported a significant improvement, and 14 % reported minimal or no change (Wright & Bifano, 1997). On the other hand, Vernon et al. divided 929 patients into two groups: a TMD group, consisting of 69 patients in whom no known cause of tinnitus was present other than one or more temporomandibular joint (TMJ) indicators (example: effect of jaw manipulation on tinnitus, incidence of pain in tinnitus ear, and sensation of fullness in tinnitus ear), and a comparison group with mixed etiologies. These two groups were then compared to determine the attributes of tinnitus that significantly separated these groups. They concluded by recommending that patients with tinnitus of unknown etiology who exhibited three or more TMJ indicators should be referred for TMD treatment (Vernon et al., 1992). Similarly, Chan and Reade reported that tinnitus may have a multifactorial etiology, similar to pain, for which the correction or elimination of any one of the factors may result in the complete resolution of symptoms (Chan & Reade, 1994). Thus, the absence of any significant or detectable auditory, genetic, drug-related, or trauma-related causes should be confirmed by otorhinolaryngologists before treating TMD patients with tinnitus.

3. Treatments for TMDs

Although the causes of TMDs have not been clarified, various treatment modalities have been clinically attempted. The most prevalent treatment is occlusal treatment, including occlusal adjustment and occlusal reconstruction. The outcomes of occlusal adjustments, in particular, have been reported several times; however, a diverse range of outcomes has been noted, from very effective to only a placebo effect (Forssel et al., 1986, 1987; Forssel et al., 1999; Kopp, 1979; Kopp & Wenneberg,1981; Tsolka et al., 1992; Tsolka & Preiskel, 1993; Vallon et al.,1991, 1995; Vallon & Nilner, 1997; Wenneberg et al., 1988). The use of occlusal adjustments has focused on the correction of a wide range of occlusal conditions (e.g., premature contact in the centric relation obtained by manipulation of the mandible, not by muscular directing; a slide between the intercuspal position [IP] and the centric relation [RCP]; and occlusal contact on the non-working side), rather than the elimination of a single condition (e.g., only premature contact in the centric relation). Thus, the results of these treatments have been difficult to interpret. Egermark-Eriksson et al. performed a long-term epidemiologic study of the relationship between occlusal factors and TMD and reported that occlusal interference, as conventionally described (in an occlusal analysis based on the reference position of the RCP obtained by manipulating the mandible), does not seem to be of much help in explaining the development or persistence of TMD (Egermark-Eriksson et al., 1987). Pullinger et al. also reported that occlusion cannot be considered the unique or dominant factor in defining TMD populations (Pullinger et al., 1993). Since the relationship between these occlusal factors (premature contact in the centric relation obtained by manipulation, not a straight slide from the centric to intercuspal position) and TMD have not been scientifically demonstrated, the Technology Conference on the Management of Temporomandibular Disorders of the NIH/NIDR (held on April 29 through May 1, 1996, in the USA) concluded that no data exists to support many commonly held beliefs regarding TMD, nor does any data exist to support the superiority of any method of management compared with the effect of a placebo. The conference participants insisted that validated diagnostic methods, with respect to sensitivity and specificity, for the identification of TMD were lacking and noted the obvious need for basic research on TMD. They then stated their belief that occlusal adjustments are invasive and that the superiority of such treatment over other non-invasive therapies has not been demonstrated in randomized controlled prospective trials. Since this conference, many conflicting opinions have been reported (Dawson, 1999; Green et al., 1998), and most clinical researchers and basic researchers have become estranged from investigations of the relationship between occlusion and TMD. Therefore, studies on occlusion and TMD have been rarely performed since that time, and treatment for TMD has shifted to more conservative modalities (Tsukiyama et al., 2001). The outcomes of these conservative treatments for TMD have been symptomatic and temporary, not resulting in a cure, because the treatments have not been applied to patients based on evidence, as the causes of TMD remain unknown. Therefore, the effects of these treatments for tinnitus have also varied (Dolowitz et al, 1964; Erlandsson et al.,1991; Parker & Chole, 1995; Principato & Barwell, 1978; Schwartz, 1956). In 2005, Torii and Chiwata reported a highly significant relationship between the TMJ sounds and the discrepancy between the habitual occlusal position (HOP) and the bite plate-induced occlusal position (BPOP) (Torii & Chiwata, 2005). TMJ sounds are the most common and most relevant sign of TMD (Könönen et al., 1993; Köhler et al., 2009; Nydell et al., 1994). Thus, the possible effect of occlusal equilibration of the BPOP on TMD signs and symptoms has also been inferred. In their study, the BPOP was defined using a physiological muscular position as a reference position. The BPOP was obtained during voluntary jaw closing, while the patient was in an upright position and after wearing an anterior bite plate for a short period time (Fig. 1).

The muscular position has been reported to vary with the posture of the subject and is thought to be less reproducible than the manually obtained centric relation (which is guided by a dentist). However, Torii and Chiwata reported that the variation in the BPOP decreased after wearing an anterior bite plate, resulting in a reduction in the severity of TMD symptoms, compared with the symptoms experienced at the beginning of treatment (Fig. 2) (Torii & Chiwata, 2010). In addition, they reported the temporary effect of a bite plate on TMD and described the need for occlusal equilibration of the BPOP (Table 1, Fig. 3).

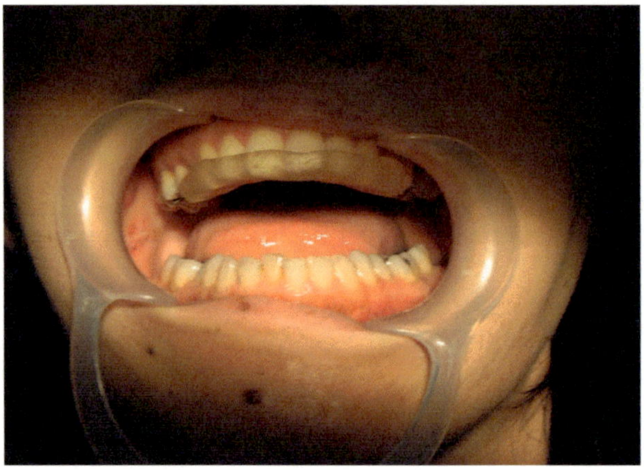

Fig. 1. **Anterior flat plane bite plate.** The plate covers the six upper anterior teeth and the first premolar teeth on both sides. The BPOP (physiological muscular position) is obtained during voluntary jaw closing after wearing the bite plate for a short period time.

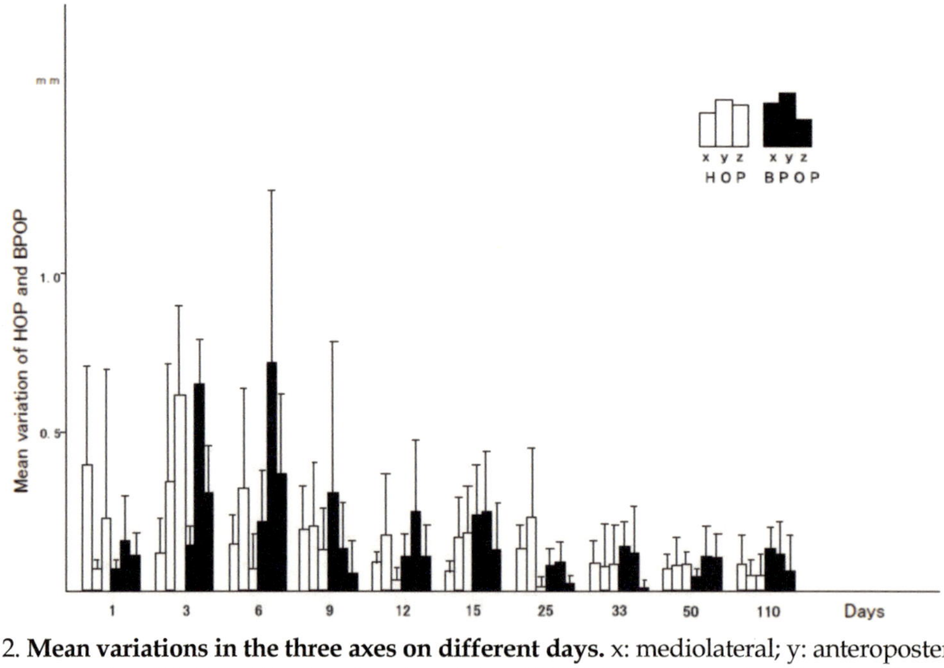

Fig. 2. **Mean variations in the three axes on different days.** x: mediolateral; y: anteroposterior; z: superoinferior. HOP: habitual occlusal position; BPOP: bite plate-induced occlusal position. This data was obtained in a case with TMJ arthralgia (Fig. 3). The symptoms disappeared 12 days after wearing an anterior flat plane bite plate.

Torii and Chiwata then performed a pilot study on the effect of occlusal equilibration using the BPOP on TMD and reported that the percentage of symptom-free patients at one year after treatment was 86% according to the Subjective Dysfunction Index (SDI) and 76% according to the Clinical Dysfunction Index (CDI); these changes in both indices after treatment were significant ($P < 0.01$) (Fig. 4 and 5) (Tables 1 and 2) (Torii & Chiwata 2010).

	After occlusal adjustment	
Occlusal discrepancy Before occlusal adjustment	No discrepancy	Discrepancy
Discrepancy	20	0
No discrepancy	1	0

McNemar's test: $X^2_{cal} = 18.05 > X^2(0.001) = 10.83$, Significant. HOP: habitual occlusal position; BPOP: bite plate-induced occlusal position.

Table 1. **Changes in the occlusal discrepancy between the HOP and BPOP before and after occlusal adjustment**

	Myofascial		Disc disp.		Arthritis	
CDI	1st Exam.	1 y	1st Exam.	1 y	1st Exam.	1 y
DiO	0%	80%	0%	86%	0%	0%
DiI	0%	20%	36%	14%	0%	100%
DiII	40%	0%	43%	0%	50%	0%
DiIII	20%	0%	21%	0%	50%	0%

CDI: Helkimo Clinical Index; 1st Exam.: first examination; 1 y: 1-year follow-up examination; Myofascial: Myofascial pain; Disc disp.: Disc displacement. DiO: no TMD; DiI: mild TMD; DiII: moderate TMD; and DiIII: severe TMD.

Table 2. **Changes in Helkimo Clinical Index at first examination and after a 1-year follow-up examination for each TMD subtype**

NS	H1 B1	H2				H6	H7			
↑ S ↓										
NS		B2	H3 B3	H4 B4	H5 B5	B6	B7	H8 B8	H9 B9	H10 B10
Days	1	3	6	9	12	15	25	33	50	110
VAS	6	3	2	2	0	0	0	0	0	0
Max.	40	42	42	42	42	42	45	45	45	45

NS: Not significant; S: Significant; Days: Days of visits; H_{1-10}: Habitual occlusal position on different day; B_{1-10}: Bite plate-induced occlusal position on different day; VAS: Score on a 10-point Visual Analogue Scale; Max.: Maximum unassisted opening (mm).

Fig. 3. **HOP and BPOP positions and TMD symptoms on different days.** The occlusal discrepancy between the HOP and the BPOP disappeared on day 6, and the disappearance was maintained between days 6 and 12. However, the discrepancy reappeared after 15 days. Therefore, equilibration of the occlusion was required to resolve the discrepancy. The occlusal equilibration was performed at 17 days.

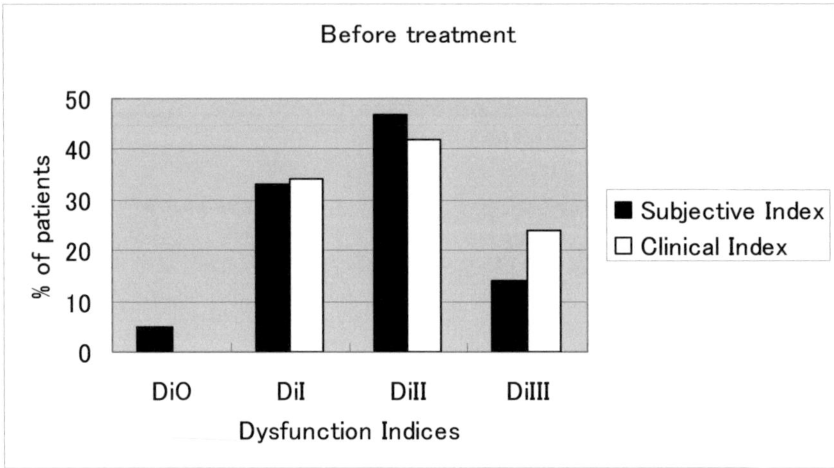

Fig. 4. **Dysfunction Index at first examination. Distribution of dysfunction indices before occlusal adjustment.** Di O: no TMD; Di I: mild TMD; Di II: moderate TMD; Di III: severe TMD.

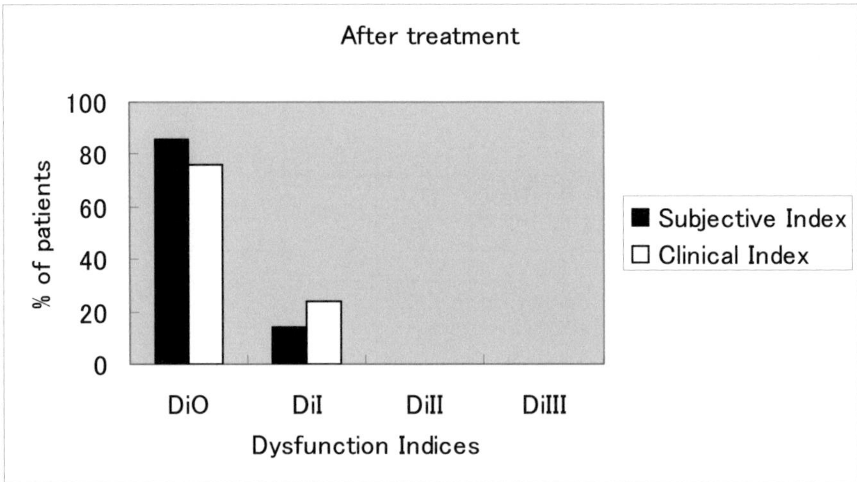

Fig. 5. **Dysfunction Index at 1-year evaluation. Distribution of dysfunction indices after occlusal adjustment.** Di O: no TMD; Di I: mild TMD; Di II: moderate TMD; Di III: severe TMD. None of the patients required an anterior bite plate during a one-year follow-up period after the completion of the occlusal adjustment. The number of visits varied between 2 and 34, with a mean of 11.0 ± 6.0 visits. Between 1 and 13 sessions of occlusal adjustment were performed, with a mean of 4.7 ± 3.5 sessions. The changes in the SDI and CDI were significant ($p<0.01$).

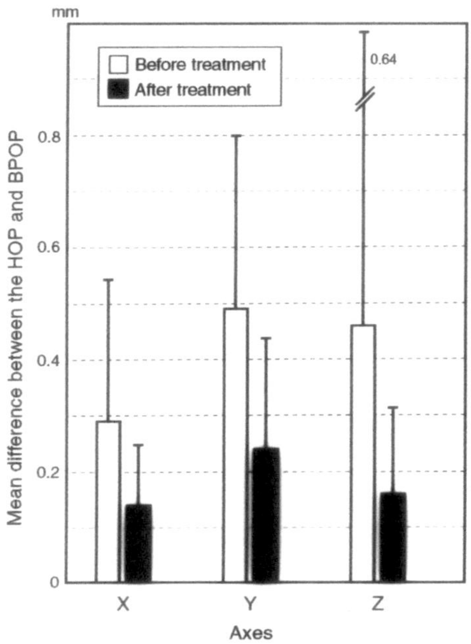

Fig. 6. **Mean HOP-BPOP difference before and after treatment.** Changes in the mean diffrence between the habitual occlusal position (HOP) and the bite plate-induced occlusal position (BPOP) before and after occlusal adjustment. x: mediolateral; y: anteroposterior; z: superoinferior. The changes were significant on the x-axis and y-axis ($p<0.05$), whereas the change on the z-axis was not significant ($p>0.1$).

Figure 6 and Table 1 indicate that a good outcome was obtained with resolution of the occlusal discrepancy by occlusal equilibration of the BPOP. Therefore, this treatment is a causal treatment, not a symptomatic treatment. In this pilot study, they reported that the otalgia of one patient and the tinnitus of another patient also completely disappeared after treatment. Table 3 shows the outcomes of the treatment of occlusal equilibration for TMDs and tinnitus in our practice.

4. Causal treatment for TMDs

Until now, occlusal discrepancy has been considered to be only one among several possible causes of TMD. At present, the only evidence-based causal treatment of TMD is occlusal equilibration, in which the habitual occlusal position (HOP) is aligned with the muscular position (BPOP). This treatment requires an articulator that can precisely reproduce the BPOP (voluntary or habitual closure movement). Torii observed various mandibular closures and found that the voluntary closing movement of the mandible consisted of a vertical movement against the occlusal plane at a point of less than 1 mm to the plane (Torii, 1989). He then developed an articulator that has a mechanism allowing vertical movement. Thus, the BPOP can be precisely reproduced using this articulator. When the upper and lower dental models are attached to the articulator with the BPOP wax record, the anteroposterior parallel space remains between both occlusal surfaces of the models after the wax record has been removed (Fig. 7).

No.	Age	Gender	Complaints	Diagnosis	Visits	Period	Outcome	Follow-up period
1.	16	M	Limited opening	Disc disp.(R)	4	2 months	resolved	5 years
			Tinnitus (R), headache				No recurrence	
2.	20	F	Limited opening	Disc disp.(B)	7	5 months	resolved	3 years
			Tinnitus(R)	Myofascial			No recurrence	
3.	22	F	Limited opening	Myofascial	16	5 months	resolved	3 years
			Headache, tinnitus(L)	Disc disp.(L)			No recurrence	
4.	28	F	Limited opening	Myofascial (L)	11	3 months	resolved	5 years
			Tinnitus (L), fullness				No recurrence	
5.	35	F	Facial pain	Myofascial (L)	4	2 months	resolved	3 years
			Headache, tinnitus (L)				No recurrence	
6.	37	F	Limited opening	Disc disp.(L)	11	3 months	resolved	10 years
			Tinnitus (L), headache				No recurrence	
7.	42	F	Facial pain	Myofascial (L)	12	2 months	resolved	5 years
			Tinnitus (L), vertigo				No recurrence	
8.	47	F	Limited opening	Disc disp.(L)	10	5 months	resolved	2 years
			Tinnitus(L)				No recurrence	
9.	73	F	TMJ pain	Arthralgia (R)	20	5 months	resolved	7 years
			Vertigo, Tinnitus (R)				No recurrence	

Table 3. **Treatment outcome of TMD patients with aural symptoms**
No: Patient number; Visits: Number of visits; Period: Treatment period. Disc Disp.: Disc displacement; Myofascial: Myofascial Pain. M: Male ; F: Female. (R), (L) and (B): Mainly affected side on the (R): right; (L): left; (B): both sides.

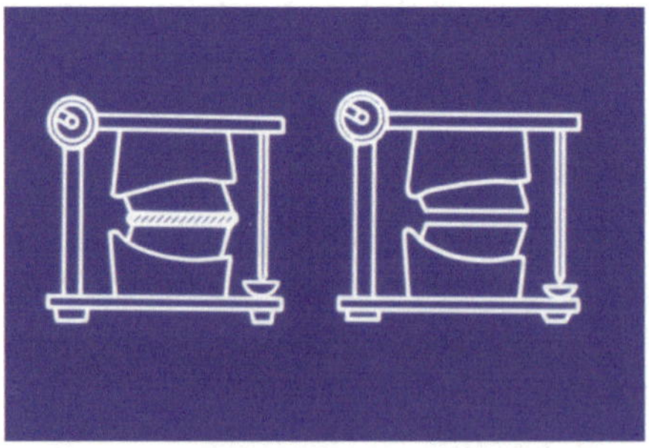

Fig. 7. **Mounting of upper and lower dental casts with BPOP wax record.** After the upper and lower casts are mounted with the BPOP wax record, and the wax record is removed, an anteroposteriorly and mediolaterally uniform space remains between both casts.

To interdigitate the teeth of the upper and lower models under this condition, a movement that is almost vertical to the occlusal plane of either model is necessary. If the models are allowed to make occlusal contact based on a hinge movement (like in a conventional articulator), the incisors and premolars make contact, and the molars will not occlude.

Therefore, to reproduce the occlusal relationship in the intercuspal position using an articulator, a mechanism that allows the upper model to be moved perpendicular to the occlusal plane is needed (Fig. 8).

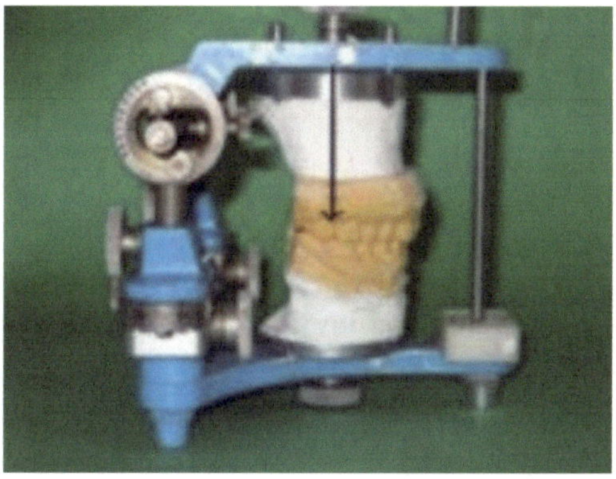

Fig. 8. **Vertically movable upper mounting ring.**

The procedure for occlusal analysis and occlusal equilibration in patients with TMDs is as follows.

1. After patient's medical history has been taken and a clinical examination has been performed, an HOP record is taken using a polysiloxane material while the patient is in an upright position. While the HOP is being recorded, the patient is asked to close his or her mouth so as to achieve maximum intercuspation and to hold that position until the material has set (approximately one minute). An anterior bite plate is then fabricated directly in the mouth using a self curing acrylic resin material; the vertical dimension should be sufficient to produce a 1.0 mm-jaw separation at the second molars. The plate should cover the upper six anterior teeth and both first premolars. The occlusal surface of the plate should be flat and perpendicular to the mandibular incisors to allow free movement in all directions. The bite plate should be worn until the severity of symptoms is resolved, usually after one or two weeks; the bite plate is worn all day except while eating, speaking, or brushing one's teeth. If the opening limitation and/or pain are not resolved using a bite plate, other symptomatic therapies, such as pharmacotherapy or physical medicine, may be necessary. Once the patient can freely open his or her mouth without pain, the treatment can proceed to the next step.
2. A BPOP record is then taken using the same material as that used to record the HOP. After the bite plate has been worn for 5 minutes, during which time the patient is asked to tap or slide his or her lower anterior teeth against the plate (muscular conditioning), the plate is removed and the recording material is applied to the occlusal surface using a syringe; the patient is then instructed to close his or her mouth until tooth contact is made and to hold that position. A BPOP wax record is then made using a wax registration material (Bite Wafer; Kerr USA, Romulus, MI, USA) and the same procedure mentioned above. The anterior part of the wafer should be cut off and softened in 60 ℃ water. After muscular conditioning using the bite plate has been performed, the softened wafer is placed on the premolars and molars on both sides. The patient is then instructed to bite the wafer gently, without biting through the wafer. The intercondylar distance is then measured using a caliper. Then, the distance between the condylar point and the lower incisal point in the occluded position is measured.

3. The intercondylar distance of the articulator is set to the same value as that of the patient. The gradation for zero on the scales on both sides indicates an intercondylar distance of 13 cm (the distance between the outsides of both condylar spheres). Therefore, when the condylar distance of the patient is 12 cm, the articulator should be reduced medially by 5 mm on each side. The articulator is then inverted, and the incisal point is marked on the mandibular cast table at a point the same distance from the condylar ball of the articulator as present in the patient. The lower cast is attached to the lower member of the articulator. The upper cast is then attached to the upper member using the BPOP wax record. At this time, a sheet of wrapping film is placed on the base of the upper cast, and some plaster is poured into the mounting ring of the upper member. The film will separate between the base of the upper cast and the poured plaster. Once the plaster has set, the film is removed and the upper cast and the poured plaster are adhered in place using α-cyanoacrylate adhesive material. This mounting method prevents dimensional changes in the mounting plaster and subsequent inaccuracies in the articulated casts.
4. Next, the occlusal discrepancy is examined. Both condylar rods of the articulator are exchanged with the analyzing rods. Recording discs attached to graph papers are then inserted into the condylar shaft. An HOP polysiloxane record is placed between the upper and lower casts and the positions are tattooed on the graph papers using colored occlusal paper with recording needles. In the same manner, the BPOP is tattooed on the same graph paper using a different color occlusal paper. The difference between the HOP and the BPOP and the direction from the BPOP to the HOP are recorded (Fig. 9).

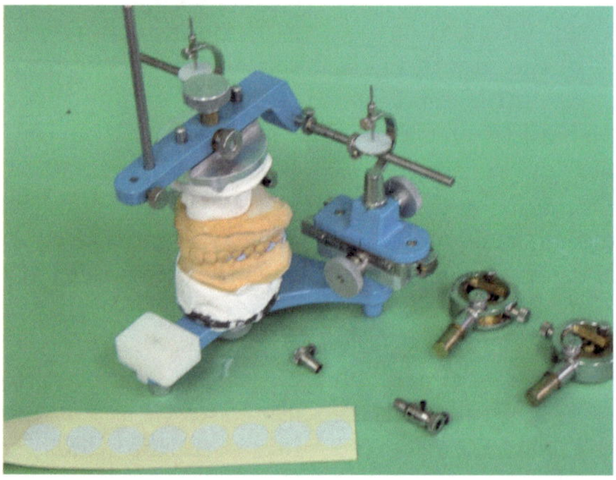

Fig. 9. **Use of the articulator as an occlusal position analyzer.**

The analyzing rods are then replaced with the condylar rods, the BPOP wax record is placed between the upper cast and the lower cast, and all the adjustable parts are set. The BPOP wax record is then removed, and the upper cast is moved downward until tooth contact has been made. Premature occlusal contact is located on the casts by marking and pulling an occlusal tape (Occlusion Foil; Coltene/Whaledent Gmbh/Co. KG, Langenau, Germany). One of several therapies (selective tooth grinding, prosthodontic and orthodontic treatments, or orthognathic surgery) may then be selected for the occlusal equilibration of the BPOP, according to the degree of the discrepancy between the HOP and the BPOP.

5. The patient should be sitting in an upright position without a headrest support. The bite plate is worn in the patient's mouth. After muscular conditioning has been performed by tapping and sliding the lower anterior teeth against the plate for 5 minutes, the plate is removed from the patient's mouth. The operator holds Miller ribbon holders (Buffalo Dental Manufacturing Co., Inc. Brooklyn, New York, USA) for the right and left quadrant recordings with red occlusal foils and asks the patient to close his or her jaw until tooth contact, then to hold that position. True occlusal contact should be confirmed by pulling the foil laterally. The premature contact should be compared with the marked contact on the casts of the articulator.
6. The premature contact on the cast is removed using a small pear-shaped carbide bur with a slow speed handpiece. The ground spot is marked with a pencil. The incisal pin of the articulator is then removed from the upper member and the articulator is closed to make occlusal contact. The incisal pin must be removed to enable a hinge movement of the articulator, because during mandibular closure, the condition in which the condyle is suspended in the capsule changes to a condition in which the condyle is contracted against the disc and the eminence, resulting in a hinge movement. The location where the next premature contact appears should be confirmed by marking and pulling with an occlusal foil. The contacts should then be recorded.
7. The patient is then reclined and the premature contact is ground down using a diamond point of a similar size and shape and a high speed handpiece. Then, the patient is raised to an upright position and the bite plate is placed in the mouth. After muscular conditioning has been performed, the patient is asked to close his or her mouth until tooth contact has been made and to mark the premature contact with an occlusal foil. If the new contact is located at the same position as on the articulator, the articulator is regarded as precisely reproducing the BPOP and it can be reliably used in the following steps during future appointments. After the new contact has been confirmed, the contact is ground down. The impressions of the upper and lower dental arches are taken in the mouth. After the patient wears the bite plate in the mouth for 5 minutes, the bite plate is removed, and a BPOP wax record is then taken for the next appointment.
8. New upper and lower casts are made and attached to the articulator in the previously described manner. Steps 6 and 7 are repeated. The occlusal adjustments are continued in the mouth by referring to the contacts marked on the casts. The occlusal adjustment is completed by confirming the occlusal contacts on the premolars and molars on both sides of the casts attached to the articulator and in the mouth. Generally, two types of premature occlusal contact occur in TMD patients: one is a premature contact at the most posterior tooth with the occlusion opened anteriorly (often seen in young patients), the other is a premature contact at the anterior tooth with the occlusion opened posteriorly (often seen in elderly patients). The former type should be treated using occlusal adjustments. The latter should be treated by restoration of the teeth or using a fixed, or removable prosthesis. After completing the occlusal equilibration, HOP and BPOP polysiloxane records are taken and both positions are confirmed to be consistent with each other on the articulator.

5. Possible mechanism of Tinnitus related to TMD

Table 3 indicates that the side affected by TMD coincides with the side affected by tinnitus. Figure 10 shows the shifts recorded on both condylar areas of the articulator in case number

9 shown in Table 3. This case has been previously reported (Torii & Chiwata, 2007). The patient complained of pain in her right ear and TMJ as well as tinnitus in her right ear. The shift on the right side was larger than that on the left side. The shifts noted after the resolution of her symptoms indicated that a displacement of the mandible from its correct position (muscular position) to a deflected position (habitual occlusal position) existed before treatment.

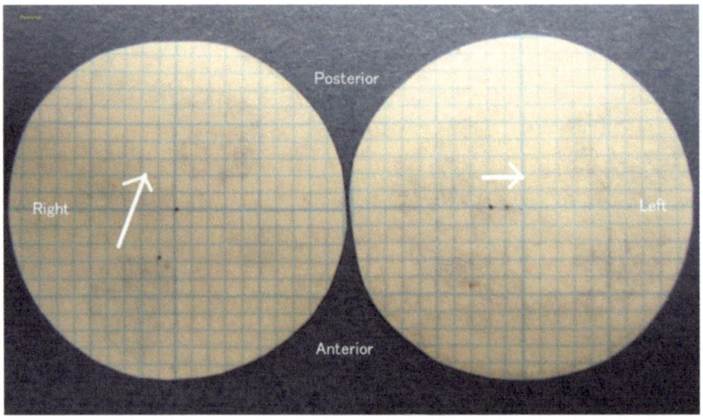

Fig. 10. **Recorded mandibular shift from the habitual occlusal position to the correct occlusal position.** In this case, the patient was diagnosed as having Méniére disease by two independent otorhinolaryngologists and was treated with isosorbide, etc. However, when the drugs failed to improve her severe symptoms, she visited our clinic complaining of pain in the right TMJ region. An occlusal analysis was performed using dental models mounted on an articulator after relieving the painful symptoms using appliance therapy, and an occlusal discrepancy was identified. Occlusal equilibration of the BPOP was then performed (see Table 3).

This displacement seems to have distorted the normal relationship between the disc and the condyle in the TMJ, since the correct relationship between the disc and the condyle is thought to be fundamentally established during the development of the function of the masticatory muscles (with regard to the muscular position, that is the BPOP) before tooth eruption. On the other hand, the existence of an occlusal discrepancy between the HOP and the BPOP means that as the mandible voluntarily closes, the elevator muscles require additional activity to adapt the mandible from the BPOP to the HOP as multiple teeth come in contact with a stable position during the change from isotonic muscle contraction to isometric. This condition may cause muscle tension, muscle fatigue and muscle spasm, resulting in muscle pain. Therefore, when considering the mechanism of tinnitus related to TMD, the displacement of the TMJ and muscle tension or spasm should be taken into account. First of all, regarding the displacement of the TMJ, Pinto found that a tiny ligament connects the neck and anterior process of the malleus to the medioposterosuperior part of the TMJ capsule, the interarticular disc, and the sphenomandibular ligament. He also described that the fibrous layer of the tympanic membrane seemed to be continuous with this tiny ligament and that the tiny ligament had an embryologic origin common with that of the malleus and incus (Pinto, 1962). However, Komori et al. performed an anatomical study and concluded that no evidence was found to support the "tiny ligament theory," as the ligament did not show any visible movement in response to a given strain. (Komori et al., 1986) Rodriguez-Vásquez et al. reported that the discomalleolar ligament is a capsular structure similar to an intrinsic ligament that is formed by the association of capsular fibers coming from the posterosuperior and medial end of the articular disc. They then described that these fibers belong to the upper lamina of the bilaminar zone (Rodríguez-Vásquez et al., 1998). Eckerdal observed the petrotympanic fissure and reported that the dimensions of the fissure and the morphologic arrangement of the intrafissural and extrafissural soft tissues do not corroborate the theory that forces generally may be conducted through the fissure from the TMJ to the ear ossicles (Eckerdal, 1991). Parker and Chole reported that although the discomalleolar ligament and the mallear portion of the sphenomandibular ligament exist and could conceivably transmit mechanical energy to the malleus, they can not account for high frequency subjective tinnitus from local perturbations of the position of the malleus (Parker & Chole, 1995). In summary, the direct transmission of force arising from the displacement of the TMJ seems unlikely to be capable of causing ear symptoms. However, Johansson et al. described in their radiographic and histologic study that a medially displaced TMJ disc may exert traction or friction or may rub against the auriculotemporal nerve trunk. Since the auriculotemporal nerve innervates the tympanic membrane, the irritation of the nerve medially or posteromedially to the TMJ, before the nerve divergence, may give rise to symptoms from the ear region (Johansson et al., 1990). Williamson reported that noxious pain stimuli to the peridiscal tissues (similar to condyle or disc displacement) could result in the constriction of the internal auditory and posterior auricular arteries. Such constriction may result in a decrease in the blood supply to the middle and inner ears. Thus, the displacement of the TMJ may cause tinnitus (Williamson, 1990). Myers reported that beginning with the appearance of a reciprocal clicking in the TMJ, the disk is forced anteromedially with full intercuspation of the teeth. This change is accompanied by the stretching of the posterior laminae and the stretching or tearing of the lateral collateral ligament. As the laminae are stretched, vascular soft tissue is pulled forward and tends to become trapped between the head of the condyle and the roof of the fossa. This injury recurs each time the teeth are intercuspated, with displacement of the disk. This causes a chronic inflammation with extension of the inflammatory area, especially along three pathways. Among these three pathways, the second pathway is located in the carotid sheath area. In the case of a displaced disk specimen, the arteries, veins and nerves are impossible to dissect because of the fibrous material adhering to them and the surrounding structures. Tension would thus be produced on the whole carotid sheath in response to any movement of the neck or jaw. This tension of the carotid sheath fibrosis would be transmitted to the jugular foramen, making the saccus endolymphaticus unable to expand to perform any possible regulation of the endolymphatic pressure; as a result, the increased endolymphatic pressure on the hair cells of the cochlea could cause tinnitus (Myers, 1988).

Regarding masticatory muscle fatigue or tension, Fuchs observed the masticatory muscle activity during sleep at night and concluded that the results of the observed activity supports the suggestion that dysfunctional patients without biteplates have a higher muscular activity during sleep than healthy persons (Fuchs, 1975). In addition, Mao et al. reported that the near absence of type II A fibers (fast-contracting, fatigue-resistant fibers) from human jaw muscles seems to suggest that these fibers may be readily susceptible to fatigue during sustained efforts at stronger force levels, since fast, fatigue-susceptible (type IIB) fibers must be recruited at these levels (Mao et al., 1993). Myrhaug reported that bite deformity is known among otologists to be a cause of tinnitus, and this type of tinnitus

arises as an autogenous vibration in the sound-conducting system, possibly because of tremor or myoclonus (myorhythmia) in the tensor muscle of the middle ear. This condition represents a fatigue reaction resulting from prolonged irritation and stress of the muscles innervated by the trigeminal nerve (masticators). This form of fatigue reaction apparently only affects the small muscles in this group because of their anatomical relationship. Hence, the two tensor muscles are in a vulnerable position in bite anomalies (Myrhaug, 1964). Koskinnen et al. and Parker and Chole were skeptical about Myrhaug's theory (Koskinnen et al., 1980; Parker & Chole, 1995). However, Watanabe et al. reported that tinnitus occurred whenever a certain mimic facial muscle contracted voluntarily or involuntarily. Under the operating microscope, the contraction of the stapedial muscle synchronous with the contraction of the mimic facial muscle was observed. The tinnitus disappeared completely immediately after the tendon of the stapedial muscle was sectioned (Watanabe et al., 1974). Myrhaug described a matter similar to that in the report of Watanabe et al. in which contractions of the tensor tympany muscle were viewed directly under a microscope during voluntary stimulation by grinning and clenching movements of the jaw.
Taking into account the facts that myofascial pain, disc displacement, tension-type headaches and tinnitus were resolved after occlusal equilibrating treatment for the BPOP (Table 3), tinnitus related to TMD may be caused by the spasmodic synkinesis of the tensor tympani and the stapedial muscle with muscle spasm of the masticatory muscles (including relative muscles), or by a decrease in the blood supply to the middle and inner ear with noxious stimuli to the peridiscal tissue, or by increased endolymphatic pressure with injury to the peridiscal tissues of the TMJ.

6. Conclusion

First, an otorhinolaryngologist should confirm the absence of any significant or detectable auditory, genetic, drug-related, or trauma-related causes of tinnitus. Then, in cases with suspected TMD, the patient should be referred to a dentist with experienced treating TMD. The dentist should perform the examination based on the RDC/TMD (Dworkin & LeResche, 1992), with particular attention to the occlusal discrepancy on an articulator. Occlusal equilibration of the BPOP should be performed to resolve the main symptoms of TMD (TMJ clicking, TMJ pain, muscle pain and difficulty in mandibular movements), since the mechanism of tinnitus related to TMD remains uncertain. Patients are fortunate if the tinnitus related to TMD disappears as a result of the treatment. In most cases, tinnitus related to TMD is likely to disappear together with the other TMD symptoms after the occlusal equilibration of the BPOP. In the absence of TMD, further medical treatments (e.g., psychiatric, neurological and otorhinolaryngological) may be indicated.

7. Acknowledgment

The author is grateful to the staff at the library of Nippon Dental University for their cooperation.

8. References

Costen, JB. (1934). A syndrome of ear and sinus symptoms dependent upon disturbed function of the temporomandibular joint. *The Annals of Otology, Rhinology & Laryngology*, Vol.43, No.1, (March 1934), pp. 1-15, ISSN 0003-4894

Costen, JB. (1936). Neuralgias and ear symptoms; associated with disturbed function of the temporomandibular joint. *The Journal of the American Medical Association,* Vol.107, No.4, (July 1936), pp. 252-255, ISSN 0022-3913

Costen, JB. (1944). Diagnosis of mandibular joint neuralgia and its place in general head pain. *The Annals of Otology, Rhinology & Laryngology* Vol.53, No.4, (December 1944), pp. 655-659, ISSN 0003-4894

Chan, SWY. & Reade, PC. (1994). Tinnitus and temporomandibular pain-dysfunction disorder. *Clinical Otolaryngology and Allied Science,* Vol.19, No.5, (October 1994), pp. 370-380, ISSN 0307-7772

Dolowitz, DA.; Ward, JW.; Fingerle, CO & Smith, CC. (1964). The role of muscular incoordination in the pathogenesis of temporomandibular joint syndrome. *Laryngoscope,* Vol.74, (June 1964), pp. 790-801, ISSN 0023-852X

Dawson, PE. (1999). Position paper regarding diagnosis, management, and treatment of temporomandibular disorders. The American Equilibration Society. *The Journal of Prosthetic Dentistry,* Vol.81, No.2, (February 1999), pp. 174-178, ISSN 0022-3913

Dworkin, SF. & LeResche L. (1992). Research diagnostic criteria for temporomandibular disorders. Review, criteria, examinations and specifications, critique. *Journal of Craniomandibular Disorders: Facial & Oral Pain,* Vol.6, No.4, (Autumn 1992), pp. 301-355, ISSN 0890-2739

Egermark-Eriksson, I.; Carlsson, GE. & Magnusson, T. (1987). A long-term epidemiologic study of the relationship between occlusal factors and mandibular dysfunction in children and adolescents. *Journal of Dental Research,* Vol.66, No.1, (January 1987), pp. 67-71, ISSN 0022-0345

Eckerdal, O. (1991). The petrotympanic fissure: a link connecting the tympanic cavity and the temporomandibular joint. *The Journal of Craniomandibular Practice,* Vol.9, No.1, (January 1991), pp. 15-22, ISSN 0886-9634

Erlandsson, SI.; Rubinstein, B. & Carlsson, SG. (1991). Tinnitus: evaluation of biofeedback and stomatognathic treatment. *British Journal of Audiology,* Vol.25, No.3, (June 1991), pp. 151-161, ISSN 0300-5364

Fuchs, P. (1975). The muscular activity of the chewing apparatus during night sleep. An examination of healthy subjects and patients with functional disturbances. *Journal of Oral Rehabilitation,* Vol.2, No.1, (January 1975), pp. 35-48, ISSN 0305-182X

Forssel, H.; Kirveskari, P. & Kangasniemi, P. (1986). Effect of occlusal adjustment on mandibular dysfunction. A double-blind study. *Acta Odontologica Scandinavica,* Vol.44, No.2, (April 1986), pp. 63-69, ISSN 0001-6357

Forssel, H.; Kirveskari, P. & Kangasniemi, P. (1987). Response to occlusal adjustment in headache patients previously treated by mock occlusal adjustment. *Acta Odontologica Scandinavica,* Vol,45, No.2 , (April 1987), pp. 77-80, ISSN 0001-6357

Forssel, H.; Kalso, E.; Koskela, P.; Vehmanen, R.; Puukka, P. & Alanen, P. (1999). Occlusal treatments in temporomandibular disorders: a qualitative systemic review of randomized controlled trials. *Pain,* Vol.83, No.3 , (December 1999), pp. 549-560, ISSN 0304-3959

Greene, CS.; Mohl, ND.; McNeill, C.; Clark, GT. & Truelove, EL. (1998). Temporomandibular disorders and science: A response to the critics. *The Journal of Prosthetic Dentistry, Vol.80,* No.2, (August 1998), pp. 214-215, ISSN 0022-3913

Johansson, AS.; Isberg, A. & Isacsson, G. (1990). A radiographic and histologic study of the topographic relations in the temporomandibular joint region: Implications for a nerve entrapment mechanism. *Journal of Oral and Maxillofacial Surgery,* Vol.48, No.9, (September 1990), pp. 953-961, ISSN 0278-2391

Kopp, S. (1979). Short-term evaluation of counseling and occlusal adjustment in patients with mandibular dysfunction involving the temporomandibular joint. *Journal of Oral Rehabilitation,* Vol.6, No.2, (April 1979) pp. 101-109, ISSN 0305-182X

Koskinnen, J.; Paavolainen, M.; Raivio, M. & Roschier, J. (1980). Otological manifestations in temporomandibular joint dysfunction. *Journal of Oral Rehabilitation,* Vol.7, No.3, (May 1980) pp. 249-254, ISSN 0305-182X

Komori, E.; Sugisaki, M.; Tanabe, H. & Kato, S. (1986). Discomalleolar ligament in the adult human. *The Journal of Craniomandibular Practice,* Vol.4, No.4, (October 1986) pp. 299-305, ISSN 0886-9634

Könönen, M. & Nyström, M. (1993). A longitudinal study of craniomandibular disorders in Finnish adolescents. *Journal of Orofacial Pain,* Vol.7, No.4, (Autumn 1993), pp. 329-336, ISSN 1064-6655

Kopp, S. & Wenneberg, B. (1981). Effects of occlusal adjustment and intra-articular injections on temporomandibular joint pain and dysfunction. *Acta Odontologica Scandinavica,* Vol.39, No.2 , (1981), pp. 87-96, ISSN 0001-6357

Köhler, AA.; Helkimo, AN.; Magnusson, T. & Hugoson, A. (2009). Prevalence of symptoms and signs indicative of temporomandibular disorders in children and adolescents. A cross-sectional epidemiological investigation covering two decades. *European Archives of Paediatric Dentistry,* Vol.10 (Suppl. 1), (November 2009) pp. 16-25, ISSN 1818-6300

McNeill C (Ed). (1990). Craniomandibular disorders. Guideline for evaluation, diagnosis, and management. Quintessence, ISBN0-86715-227-3, Chicago

Myrhaug, H. (1965). The incidence of ear symptoms in cases of malocclusion and temporomandibular joint disturbances. *The British Journal of Oral Surgery,* Vol.2, No.1, (July 1964), pp. 28-32, ISSN 0007-117X

Myers, LJ. (1988). Possible inflammatory pathways relating temporomandibular joint dysfunction to otic symptoms. *The Journal of Craniomandibular Practice,* Vol.6, No.1, (January 1988), pp. 64-70, ISSN 0886-9634

Mao, J.; Stein, RB. & Osborn, JW. (1993). Fatigue in human jaw muscles: a review. *Journal of Orofacial Pain,* Vol.7, No.2, (Spring 1993), pp. 135-142, ISSN 1064-6655

Nydell, A.; Helkimo, M. & Koch G. (1994). Craniomandibular disorders in children - A critical review of the literature. *Swedish Dental Journal,* Vol.18, No.5, (1994), pp. 191-205, ISSN 0347-9994

Pinto, OF. (1962). A new structure to the temporomandibular joint and middle ear. *The Journal of Prosthetic Dentistry,* Vol.12, No.1, (January-February 1962), pp. 95-103, ISSN 0022-3913

Principato, JJ. & Barwell, DR. (1978). Biofeedback training and relaxation exercises for treatment of temporomandibular joint dysfunction. *Otolaryngology,* Vol.86, No.5, (September-October 1978), pp. 766-769, ISSN 0161-6439

Pullinger, AG.; Seligman, DA. & Gornbein, JA. (1993). A multiple logistic regression analysis of the risk and relative odds of temporomandibular disorders as a function of

common occlusal features. *Journal of Dental Research*, Vol.72, No.6, (June 1993), pp. 968-979, ISSN 0022-0345
Parker, WS. & Chole, RA. (1995). Tinnitus, vertigo, and temporomandibular disorders. *American Journal of Orthodontics and Dentofacial Orthopedics*, Vol.107, No.2, (February 1995), pp. 153-158, ISSN 0889-5406
Rubinstein, B. (1993). Tinnitus and craniomandibular disorders: Is there a link? *Swedish Dental Journal*, Vol.95(Suppl), (1993), pp. 1-46, ISSN 0348-6672
Rodríguez-Vásquez, JF.; Mérida-Velasco, JR.; Mérida-Velasco, JA. & Jiménez-Collado, J. (1998). Anatomical considerations on the discomalleolar ligament. *Journal of Anatomy*, Vol.192, No.4, (May 1998), pp. 617-621, ISSN 0021-8782
Sicher, H. (1948). Temporomandibular articulation in mandibular over-closure. *The Journal of the American Dental Association*, Vol.36, No.2, (February 1948), pp. 131-139, ISSN 0002-8177
Schwartz, LL. (1956). A temporomandibular joint pain dysfunction syndrome. *Journal of Chronic Diseases*, Vol.3, No.3, (March 1956), pp. 284-293, ISSN 0021-9681
Tsolka, P.; Morris, RW. & Preiskel, HW. (1992). Occlusal adjustment therapy for craniomandibular disorders: A clinical assessment by a double-blind method. *The Journal of Prosthetic Dentistry*, Vol.68, No.6, (December 1992), pp. 957-964, ISSN 0022-3913
Tsolka, P. & Preiskel, HW. (1993). Kinesiographic and electromyographic assessment of the effects of occlusal adjustment therapy on craniomandibular disorders by a double-blind method. *The Journal of Prosthetic Dentistry*, Vol69, No.1, (January 1993), pp. 85-92, ISSN 0022-3913
Torii, K. (1989). Analysis of rotation centers of various mandibular closures. *The Journal of Prosthetic Dentistry*, Vol.61, No.3, (March 1989), pp. 285-291, ISSN 0022-3913
Tsukiyama, Y.; Baba, K. & Clark, GT. (2001). An evidence-based assessment of occlusal adjustment as a treatment for temporomandibular disorders. *The Journal of Prosthetic Dentistry*, Vol.86, No.1, (July 2001), pp. 57-66, ISSN 0022-3913
Torii, K. & Chiwata, I. (2005). Relationship between habitual occlusal position and flat bite plane-induced occlusal position in volunteers with and without temporomandibular joint sounds. *The Journal of Craniomandibular Practice*, Vol. 23, No.1, (January 2005), pp. 16-21, ISSN 0886-9634
Torii, K. & Chiwata, I. (2007). Occlusal management for a patient with aural symptoms of unknown etiology: a case report. *Journal of Medical Case Reports*, 2007,1:85, Available from
http://www.jmedicalcasereports.com/content/1/1/85
Torii, K. & Chiwata, I. (2010). Occlusal adjustment using the bite plate-induced occlusal position as a reference position for temporomandibular disorders: a pilot study. *Head & Face Medicine*, 2010;6:5, Available from
http://www.head-face-med.com/content/6/1/5
Torii, K. & Chiwata, I. (2010). A case report of the symptom-relieving action of an anterior flat plane bite plate for temporomandibular disorder. *The Open Dentistry Journal*, 2010;4:218-222, Available from
http://www.benthamscience.com/open/todentj/index.htm

Vallon, D.; Ekberg, EC.; Nilner, M. & Kopp, S. (1991). Short-term effect of occlusal adjustment on craniomandibular disorders including headaches. Acta Odontologica Scandinavica, Vol.49, No.2, (April 1991), pp. 89-96, ISSN 0001-6357

Vernon, J.; Griest, S. & Press, L. (1992). Attributes of tinnitus that may predict temporomandibular joint dysfunction. *The Journal of Craniomandiblar Practice,* Vol.10, No.4, (October 1992), pp. 282-287, ISSN 0886-9634

Vallon, D.; Ekberg, EC.; Nilner, M. & Kopp, S. (1995). Occlusal adjustment in patients with craniomandibular disorders including headaches. A 3- and 6-month follow-up. *Acta Odontologica Scandinavica,* Vol.53, No.1, (February 1995), pp. 55-59, ISSN 0001-6357

Vallon, D. & Nilner, M. (1997). A longitudinal follow-up of the effect of occlusal adjustment in patients with craniomandibular disorders. *Swedish Dental Journal,* Vol.21, No.3, (1997), pp. 85-91, ISSN 0347-9994

Watanabe, I.; Kumagami, H. & Tsuda, Y. (1974). Tinnitus due to abnormal contraction of stapedial muscle. *Journal for Oto-Rhino-Laryngology and its related specialties,* Vol.36, No.4, (1974), pp. 217-226, ISSN 0301-1569

Williamson, EH. (1990). The interrelationship of internal derangements of the temporomandibular joint, headache, vertigo, and tinnitus: A survey of 25 patients. *The Journal of Craniomandibular Practice,* Vol.8, No.4, (October 1990), pp. 301-306, ISSN 0886-9634

Wright, EF. & Bifano, SL. (1997). Tinnitus improvement through TMD therapy. *The Journal of the American Dental Association,* Vol.128, No.10, (October 1997), pp. 1424-1432, ISSN 0002-8177

Wenneberg, B.; Nystrom, T. & Carlsson, GE. (1998). Occlusal equilibration and other stomatognathic treatment in patients with mandibular dysfunction and headache. *The Journal of Prosthetic Dentistry,* Vol.59, No.4, (April 1988), pp. 478-483, ISSN 0022-3913

3

Tinnitus and a Linked Stomatognathic System

Luis Miguel Ramirez Aristeguieta
Universidad de Antioquia, Medellin
Colombia

1. Introduction

Most patients associate tinnitus (false sound perception) with desperation and a Sui genereis awareness. Normally, it is accompanied by another otic symptoms that worse the aversive experience. For some individuals, tinnitus occupied the majority of their attention cosmos by negative cognitive-emotional conditioning. People that suffer this condition have a considerable work-familiar-individual challenge. It also, could be shared with additional varied otic and cranial symptoms like otic fullness, otalgia, hearing loss, dizziness, and a diffuse craniofacial and stomatognathic (chewing machinery) pain with a diffuse presentation (headaches, mialgia arthralgia and cervicalgia).[1]
Traditionally, tinnitus origin has been linked to conductive, sensorial or both mixed otic origins. A nervous dysfunction explanation has more adherences in the health community. With this in mind, a sensorineuronal tinnitus dysfunction has been understood as triggered by sound energy transmission complications with peripheral or central nerve damage origins. Lately, the health community has commenced understanding how a stomatognathic's (conductive) scenario has shown evidence of their links.
In this chapter the reader is invited to ingoing into an stimulating and almost new form of looking tinnitus aetiology (among other otic referred symptoms) based in the research with some biological models that permit to analyse a variety of pathophysiological tinnitus associations with the chewing apparatus.
In this sense, it must be first comprehended that the stomatognathic structure must be fatigued and in a dysfunctional state to produce tinnitus and other referred otic symptoms. This state in which the stomatognathic musculoskeletal system is hyper-functional, tender and exhausted is known as temporomandibular disorders (TMD). TMD can generate referred craniofacial symptomatology (where origin differed form its real location) that involves not only the auditive system and take influence in cervical and cranial diffuse discomfort too.
Thirty years after Costen[2] (1934) pioneering ideas about otic referred symptoms starting from the stomatognathic system, Myrhaug[3] affirmed that the middle ear belong to the chewing system although it served the auditory system. Unfortunately for these otolaryngologists this logic was advanced for their time and was considered almost a heretic concept receiving an unjust opposition by their own medical community. Trying to rescue these clever researchers contributions some analysis about the otic/chewing linking connections will be developed.
There are fourteen possible stomatognathic models (among embryological, musculoskeletal, ligamental, vascular and neural) that offer adequate explanations for tinnitus and other

linked otic-cranio-cervico-facial referred symptoms.[4,5,6] This analysis equally tries to support actual evidence about otic referred symptoms reliefs by stomatognathic therapeutic.[7] Nowadays, there is no doubt that a multidisciplinary approach (otolaryngology, odontology, neurology including another health disciplines) is essential for an assertive diagnosis, treatment and prognosis of this particular symptomatology.

2. Dysfunctional stomatognathic system and Bruxism

Temporomandibular disorders (TMD) consist of musculoskeletal pain conditions, characterized by pain in the temporomandibular joint (TMJ) and/or mastication muscles. This condition involves a wide range of craniofacial conditions having multiple origins that produces a large variety of non-objective signs and symptoms.[8] These could be primary, referred or combined from cervical muscles and associated cranial structures and appear similarly in adults, as well as, in children [9,10]. The prevalence of TMD is 1.5 to 4 times more common in women than in men.[11] After low back pain, TMD occupied the second place of musculoskeletal disability condition.

The etiology of the TMD can be isolated or the combination of macrotrauma and microtrauma (Bruxism) and this last appears to play a significant role in TMD and craniofacial referred symptoms.[12] Bruxism is an intense and subconscious rhythmic motor activity of non-functional teeth grinding and clenching. Besides exceeding the structural tolerance of the biological tissues, it triggers a cascade of primary and referred symptomatology (Figure 1).[13,14,15,16,17]

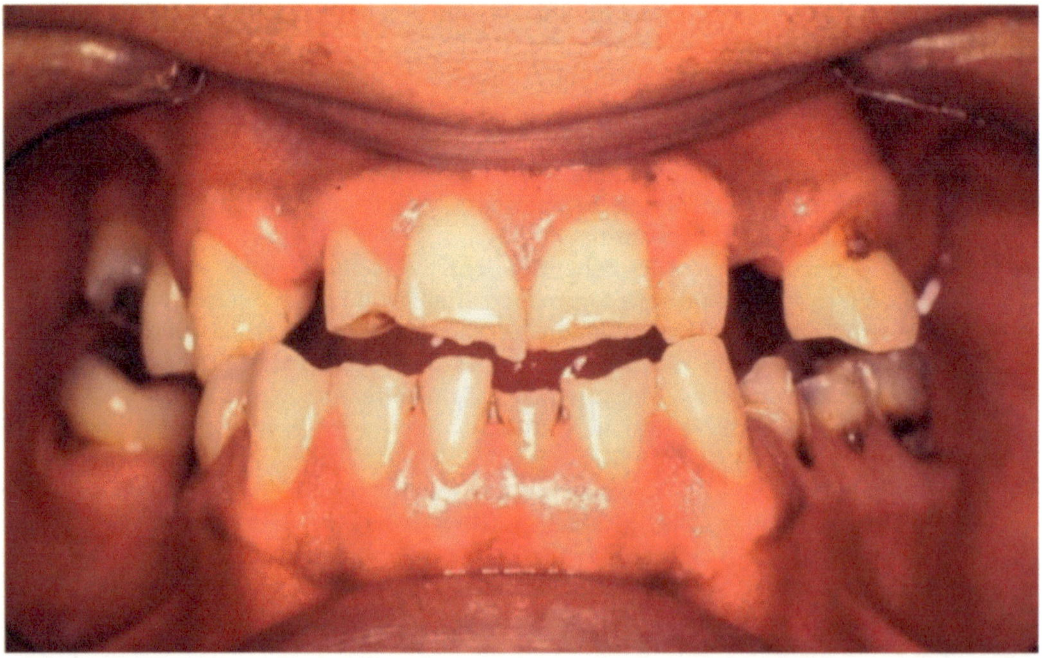

Fig. 1. Grinding effects on teeth due to bruxism in a 45-year male patient. Consequently with his deteriorate teeth appearance; an advanced primary and referred musculoskeletal symptomatology is manifest. Photography use authorized to the author (Patient's record).

3. Stomatognathic referred otic symptoms

Since almost a century, health literature has closely perceived otic symptoms and other craniofacial complaints in TMD. However, there is little evidence for an association between the two. An integrated biological basis for otic symptoms in TMD is presented from both anatomical and physiological points of view. To accomplish a central-peripheral mechanisms involved, they are discussed along the chapter. Basic sciences let integrate diverse point of views in the understanding of common symptoms. This matter deals with perspectives of otic symptoms triggered or exacerbated by atypical stomatognathic dynamics.[18,19]

Otic symptoms include otalgia, tinnitus, vertigo-dizziness, subjective hearing loss, and otic fullness.[20,21,22,23,24,25] Such otic symptoms evidently can be originated in the auditory system (as a primary symptom) but are also habitually a symptom of an associated neighboured stomatognathic dysfunction (secondary or referred symptom).

Otic symptoms related to the masticatory system can be found in both adult and paediatric populations.[26] Monson and Wright (1920) related the position of the TMJ to hearing impairment and in 1925, Decker also related otic symptoms to stomatognathic TMJ. Costen in 1934 associated otic symptoms later named Costen's syndrome.[27,28] Although the literature supports a connection between otic symptoms and TMD; it is still an open question as to whether this association is causal or accidental.[29] A screening search permit to observe apparent correlations between otic symptoms and TMD in some studies from 1933 to 2011 (Table 1).[30,31,32,33,34,35,36,37,38,39,40,41,42,43,44,45,46,47,48,49,50,51,52,53,54,55,56,57,58,59,60,61,62,63,64,65,66]

Overall, 12.732 TMD patients were mentioned in n=54 articles. Otalgia was present in 50.9 % of the patients (n=44), tinnitus in 39.1 % (n=47), otic fullness in 44 % (n=24), vertigo in 30.3 % (n=39), and hearing loss in 24.4 % (n=28). Salvetti et al.[67] found that the prevalence of otic symptoms in the general population varied from 10% to 31% and increase to 85% in TMD patients.

Taking this in mind, a relationship between otic symptoms and TMD have been found since the beginning of the last century, with some interesting findings: Kuttila et al.[46] found a prevalence of tinnitus (12-17%), otalgia (12-16%), and otic fullness (5-9%) in subjects with TMD. According to Rubinstein[68] 33-67% of TMD patients reported tinnitus. Gelb et al.[22] found that 42% of patients with TMD reported tinnitus, 35% reported otalgia, 18% reported dizziness, and 14% reported hearing loss. Besides, Cooper et al.[21] found 40-70% of TMD patients experiencing dizziness and 5-40% feeling vertigo. Lam et al.[69] noted in a retrospective work that 26.4% of TMD patients had otic symptoms with a prevalence of tinnitus higher than that found in the general population. Bjorne and Agerberg[70] proved that Meniere's disease (understood as hearing loss, frequently associated with tinnitus, otic fullness, and paroxistic vertigo) is strongly related to TMD symptoms.

Recently, the somatic modulation capacity on tinnitus has served to evidence a potential connection. Lockwood et al.[71] found that up to 75% of subjects were able to vary tinnitus intensity by clenching the jaw, increasing digital cranial muscle pressure, and moving the eyes (gaze-evoked tinnitus). Vernon et al. ([72]) although expressed no association between tinnitus from TMJ origins; observed increased intensity of tinnitus when jaw-clenching or other jaw movements occurred. Levine[73] found that tinnitus can be modulated by isometric oro-facial and cranio-cervical manipulations.

In addition to the pain dimension, Hazell[74] reported 39% of patients suffering from tinnitus with frequent tension headaches with fatigue and muscle soreness in the facial and

Authors	N° TMD patients	% otalgia	% tinnitus	% vertigo	% hearing loss	% otic fullness
Goodfriend 1933 (30) Ʊ	91	3	14	5	26	---
Costen 1934 (2) Ʊ	400	38	13	12	13	6
Gelb-Arnold 1959 (24) Ʊ	100	13	27	5	---	---
Kelly-Goodfriend 1960 (51) Ʊ	102	---	---	75,5	---	---
Kelly-Goodfriend 1964 (52) Ʊ	105	25	44	100	44	30,4
Myrhaug 1964 (3) Ʊ	1391	21	32	28	32	---
Dolowitz *et al.*, 1964 (115) Ʊ	66	100	43	5	38	48
Gelb *et al.*, 1967 (23) Ʊ	742	36	40	20	15	---
Bernstein *et al.*, 1969 (20) Ʊ	86	93	42	14	33	62
Sharav *et al.*, 1978 (118) Ʊ	42	---	---	23	---	---
Principato-Barwell 1978 (50) Ʊ	25	100	44	44	---	---
Koskinen *et al.*, 1980 (45) Ʊ	47	47	20	26	24	26
Brookes *et al.*, 1980 (33) Ʊ	45	82	76	33	80	62
Carlsson et al. 1982 (37) ¥	350	38	15	17	15	---
Gelb-Bernstein 1983 (41) Ʊ	1142	---	41,5	20,6	15,4	---
Gelb-Bernstein 1983 (42) Ʊ	200	---	36	40	24,5	48
Fricton *et al.*, 1985 (40) Ʊ	164	42	42	23	17,7	---
Cooper *et al.*, 1986 (22) Ʊ	476	50	36	40	38	---
Wedel-Carlsson 1986 (53) Ʊ	148	---	14	15	14	---
Bush 1986 (35) Ʊ	105	82	33	---	---	---
Bush 1987 (36) Ʊ	35	---	33	---	---	---
Williamson 1990 (153) Ʊ	25	---	---	44	---	---
Henderson *et al.*, 1992 (119) Ʊ	21	85,7	90,5	76,1	66,6	90,5
Chole-Parker 1992 (38) ¥	338	100	59	70	---	---
Vernon *et al.*, 1992 (72) ¥	69	45	100	---	---	75
Cooper *et al.*, 1993 (21) Ʊ	996	63	51	41	25	30
Ogutcen-Toller *et al.*, 1993 (114) Ʊ	57	40	17	8,7	26	5
Ciancaglini *et al.*, 1994 (39) Ʊ	797	1.6	6.4	1.6	7,6	---
Ren-Isberg 1995 (169) ¥	53	98,1	100	54,7	---	92,5
Parker-Chole 1995 (49) ¥	338	100	59	70	---	---
Keersmaekers *et al.*, 1996 (25) Ʊ	400	42	---	---	---	---
Manni *et al.*, 1996 (48) Ʊ	53	33,9	22,6	33,9	7,5	41,5
Wright *et al.*, 1997 (170) Ʊ	93	38	38	---	---	---
Karjalainen *et al.*, 1997 (34) ¥	63	13	---	3	---	---
Luz *et al.*,, 1997 (47) Ʊ	894	10,8	---	3,1	---	---
Watanabe et al., 1998 (55) Ʊ	143	---	15	10	---	11
de Felicio *et al.*, 1999 (58) ¥	30	53,3	66,6	20	20	76,6
Kuttila *et al.*, 1999 (46) Ʊ	411	14	15	---	---	7
D'Antonio *et al.*, 2000 (57) Ʊ	90	100	51,1	31,1	---	---
Wright *et al.*, 2000 (56) Ʊ	15	15	14	11	---	---
Bruto *et al.*, 2000 (65) Ʊ	40	75	17,5	---	15	17,5
Lam *et al.*, 2001 (69) Ʊ	470	32	26	18	12	---
Pascoal et al 2001 (66) Ʊ	126	50	50	34	10	52
Peroz 2001 (85) Ʊ	221	37	3.8	---	---	---
Tuz et al 2003 (54) Ʊ	200	57,2	48,3	42,7	29,4	---
de Felicio et al 2004 (59) Ʊ	27	59,2	74	---	---	74,1
Sobhy et al 2004 (86) Ʊ	30	56,7	20	---	---	---
Bernhardt et al., 2004 (18) ¥	30	---	30	---	19	---
Kaygusuz et al. 2006 (44)	44	31,8	18,2	13,6	6,8	13,6
Abou-Atme et al. 2006 (32)	530	19,6	---	---	---	26,7
De Felicio et al., 2008 (60) ¥	20	65	60	---	---	90
De Felicio et al., 2010 (61) ¥	30	13,4	8,8	---	---	13,5
Pekkan et al., 2010 (63) ¥	25	72	52	20	8	56
Bernhardt et al., 2011 (64) ¥	191	---	12,6	---	---	---
Media		50,9	39,1	30,3	24,4	44,0
Total	12732					
n	54	44	47	39	28	24

Ʊ Clinical not controlled studies
¥ Epidemiological / Controlled studies

Table 1. Different TMD patient populations suffering referred otic symptoms.

masticatory muscles. Kuttila et al.[75] showed how otic fullness, earaches, shoulder and TMD pain are risk factors for recurrent tinnitus.
TMD appear to play a relevant participation role in otic referred symptoms without misestimating another potential origins within and outside the auditory system, including viral cranial neuropathy, intracranial vascular anomalies, cerebrovascular disease, cardiovascular disease, mediastinal tumours, Meniere's disease, ear and head trauma, chronic myringitis, impacted cerumen, otic infections, ototoxic drugs, acoustic neuroma, multiple sclerosis, neuroplastic changes, noise exposure, otosclerosis, and presbycusis. In this sense, a multifactorial cause with wide cranio-cervico-facial structure participation should carefully be considered in a teamwork effort with an exclusionary diagnostic approach.
How TMD affect the auditory system must be understood in different evidence levels. A morphologic-embryologic-neurophysiologic way could help to understand the pathophysiology of these clinical events. However, clinicians should be made aware that a single cause of otic symptoms competes with a multifactorial origin. Over the last few years, the most acknowledged clarifying models have focused on central nervous system (CNS) networks. However, peripherally structures could be also an important issue to view regarding the aetiology of otic referred symptoms. An integral model concerning neurological, anatomical and physiological perspectives offer a wider angle for the multiple and dynamic enlightenments linking TMD and otic symptoms.

4. Neural explanations

Some otic experiences like tinnitus, hearing loss, vertigo, and otalgia can be explained from a multidimensional neurological point of view. Most investigators have focused on tinnitus by the multiple CNS interconnections and plasticity that actually occur.

4.1 First neural exploration

Symptoms such as vertigo, tinnitus, and subjective hearing loss can result from an auditory innervation pattern involving the trigeminal nerve. Vass et al.[76] found that trigeminal vascular system innervation in guinea pigs controls cochlear and vestibular labyrinth function. This plays an important role in regulating and balancing cochlear vascular tone and vestibular labyrinth channel and may be responsible for the symptomatic complexity of some cochlear diseases related to inner ear blood flow. Trigeminal ophthalmic fibre projection to the cochlea through the basilar and anterior inferior cerebellar arteries may play an important role in vascular tone in quick and vasodilatatory responses to intense noise. Inner ear diseases that produce otic symptoms such as sudden hearing loss, vertigo, and tinnitus can originate from reduced cochlear blood flow due to the presence of abnormal activity in the trigeminal ganglion, which is possible in patients with herpes zoster, migraines and TMD. A parallel discovery by Shore et al.[77] found that the trigeminal ganglion innervates and modulates the vascular supply of the ventral and dorsal portions of the cochlear nucleus and the superior olivary complex.

4.2 Second neural exploration

Levine et al.[78] suggested that a somatic auditory perception interference in the dorsal cochlear nucleus (DCN) and ventral cochlear nucleus by trigeminal innervation and named it "somatic tinnitus". [78,79] Shore et al.[80] found this connectivity in the superior olivary complex (involved in sound localisation and centrifuge reflex). Such trigeminal-auditory neural communication may cause a significant impact on the neurons from this nucleus, interfering with the auditory pathway (tinnitus), which is directed towards the auditory cortex in the presence of constant peripheral somatic signals from ophthalmic and mandibular trigeminal peripheral innervation. Young et al.[81] affirm that such a stimulus is so strong that it can interfere with moderate-level acoustic stimuli.[82] The perception originates from mechano-sensory and in a minor amount from nociceptive spinal and cranial nerve impulses in the caudal spinal nucleus and is modulated by muscle fatigue in the head and neck areas. CNS interaction between the somatosensory system and multilevel auditory tracts (including the inferior colliculus and extralemniscal auditory pathway is a fundamental property of the auditory system.[83] Trigeminal somatosensory input to the inferior colliculus employs the same DCN pattern (bimodal inhibition-excitation synapses) as a reflection of its multimodal integration. Somatosensory input in TMD may explain the origin of otic symptoms such as subjective hearing loss and tinnitus when no disease is within the hearing organ.[84,85,86]

Kaltenbach et al.[87] proposed a tinnitus model in which hyperactive neurons in the DCN can undergo different forms of plasticity (temporal, by injury, by somatosensory modulation, and by activity-dependent stimulus), becoming an important contributor to producing and modulating tinnitus depending on DCN neuron cellular membrane dynamics. Developing DCN hyperactivity seems to depend on the balance of excitatory and inhibitory input, showing that the auditory system is not an electrically peaceful system. Shore and Zhou[80] found that 70% of the DCN has a bimodal sensorial pattern consisting of approximately 2/3 suppressive 1/3 enhancing integrations. Zhou and Shore[88] and Kaltenbach[89] explained the possible function that these neural auditive and somatosensory network interactions may accomplish in the DCN. The somatosensory role of the direct or indirect neuronal network interactions in producing and modulating tinnitus has suggested that numerous inputs to the cochlear nuclear complex is a possible proprioceptive information mechanism from the spinal trigeminal nucleus amongst other nuclear complex inputs (gracile, cuneatus, reticular system, vestibular). Such proprioceptive information mechanisms are necessary for vocalisation-communication (vocal structures position), for body situation, and for pursuing a sound source (pinna position) in the eye-to-head and head-to-space orientation, which is important in environmental alerting. This neuronal network has been suggested as being a possible autogenous sound eradication mechanism, suppressing self-produced (autogenous) sounds (chewing, self-vocalisation and respiration). Kaltenbach[89] correspondingly showed that the DCN is an integral part of the brainstem's circuits and is essential in biphasically auditory stimuli attention (projection recipient and source) interconnecting segmental structures (locus ceruleus, reticular formation). The objective of this sensorineuronal attention system is to coordinate the origin of auditory stimuli for the head, eyes, and ears. Taking this in mind, it should be recalled that the middle ear stapedius and tensor tympani muscles' auditive protective and discriminative ability, together with "Kaltenbach's attention model" during a centrifuge reflex, is also important as a normal conductive selective attention (discriminative) system.

4.3 Third neural exploration

It appears that sensorineuronal tinnitus is an altered neural activity effect and may result from a lesion or dysfunction at any level of the auditory system. Tinnitus can be centrally triggered by several mechanisms: auditory nerve transaction, vascular compression, exposure to intense sound, and/or ototoxic drugs (i.e. cisplatin, among others). Reduced auditory-nerve input (hearing loss or deafness) reduces inhibition of the DCN and spontaneously enhances central auditory pathway motion, which is experienced as tinnitus; however, some tinnitus patients do not present any trauma history, hearing loss or deafness. Corresponding, a lack of DCN inhibition can also be modulated by somatosensory (TMD) input without cortical or sub-cortical inhibition.[78,79]

Lockwood et al.[90] consider this DCN inhibition phenomenon as being a failure of normal "cross-modal inhibition" and suggested that hearing loss causes pathways to become reorganised by neuroplasticity in the central auditory system. This leads to abnormal interactions between auditory and other central somatosensory pathways. They proved that cortical tinnitus explains an interesting scenario in which the origin of tinnitus is more complex due to false sensory perception parallel levels (from peripheral biphasic to cerebral cortex levels). Information in the auditory pathways does not solely flow from the ear to the brain; there is also considerable flow in the opposite direction mediating and filtering human auditory system gain. Jeanmonod et al.[91] proved that the thalamic relay synapses explains that rhythmic discharges in the cortex are due to signal loops by thalamic lack of inhibition causes this phantom sound to be integrated in a multidimensional aetiological viewpoint. Unbalanced excitatory and inhibitory signals in the multimodal non-specific thalamic nucleus with reverberating thalamo-cortico-thalamo loops may produce tinnitus in the auditory cortex.

Cacace[92] stated that association cortical areas (including Wernicke's area) are of prime importance in receiving multilevel segmental cross-modal interactions between auditory, somatosensory, somatomotor, and limbic system areas and tracts which do not exclusively involve peripheral auditory input in perceiving subjective sounds. Cacace stated that there is natural cortical concurrence of different perceptual sensorial experiences (synesthesia), which combines several modalities and may explain tinnitus in other primary cross-modal cortical area integration that would involve pain (TMD). Muhlnickel et al.[93] hypothesised a plastic reorganisation of the tonotopic cortical map, which might present tinnitus in cochlear hair cell loss (subjective hearing loss) as being a phantom phenomenon such as with phantom limb pain in the somatosensorial cortex. Such cortical reorganisation might also begin from on-going tinnitus.

4.4 Fourth neural exploration

Behavioural dimension of tinnitus is equally important, as are emotional, cognitive and attentional models regarding pain (inhibition or facilitation) and also rhythmic oromotor activity (bruxism).[94,95] This behavioural dimension is modulated by cortical (amygdala, cingulate, insular cortex, etc.) and subcortical levels (reticular system, locus ceruleus, etc.). Tinnitus may produce different effects on each person's social, emotional, and physical aspects, due to the level of annoyance produced by it (de-compensation).[96] Attention and affective components of tinnitus anxiety and phobias emerge in the limbic system; moreover, the psychosocial dimension may trigger tinnitus states. Such broad limbic organisation is the most important CNS modulator component that is able to transform (positively or negatively) the whole organism's homeostasis (pain, concentration, temperature, muscle activity, memory, motivation, autonomous tonicity, hormonal and endocrine balance, feed, sleep, and other circadian rhythms) as a response to survival instinct stimulus. Mild tinnitus could be someone's worst experience (high priority attention) but also the least significant incident (low priority attention) for the same person and depending on personal bio-psycho-social reaction and its negative emotional reinforcement. Curiously, these symptom limbic frontiers triggered and modulated by the cognitive-behavioural dimension are transited in a similar way for bruxistic episodes that share common territories with apparently different multilevel effects.

Kaltenbach[89] explained that reciprocal DCN connections to subcortical limbic system structures relating to anxiety stimulate the locus ceruleus and during depression state the raphe nuclear complex. Serotonergic raphe nuclear complex activity is associated with the presence of tinnitus (increased serotonin levels) and depression (lower serotonin levels). Moreover, locus ceruleus is a multifunctional noradrenergic neuronal conformation serving many reflexes and having crucial emotional limbic component work. Fascinatingly, the same limbic system, which interacts with the DCN, also intermingles with the trigeminal motor nucleus producing bruxism and a TMD effect. Kato et al.[94] stated that bruxism is an intense, spontaneous, rhythmic motor manifestation, secondary to a sequence of autonomic physiological changes expressed in accelerated heart rate and increased motor, cortical, and breathing activity, which precede bruxism stages. Such rhythmic muscular dysfunctional episodes are triggered in attention-affective stressful conditions, which seem to concomitantly initiate tinnitus. Anxiety and depression thus appear to cause otic symptoms in a varied CNS structure.

5. Embryological explanation

TMJ development and other neighbouring structures in humans (such as pharynx, Eustachian tube, and tympanic cavity) is complex and continues to be investigated.[97] The mandible is formed from the ventral part of Meckel's cartilage, which is the first branchial arch.[98] The oscicles (malleus, incus, and partially the stapes) are formed from the dorsal part of Meckel's cartilage and Reichert's cartilage (second branchial arch). The malleus has a double origin in these oscicles; the anterior process originates from mesenchymal cells (os goniale), through intramembranous ossification, and the rest form from Meckel's cartilage, through endochondral ossification[99,100] The malleus is related to the TMJ (condylar and temporal blastemas) by fibrous connections (lateral pterygoid muscle) passing through the petrotympanic fissure, which Rees named the discomalleolar ligament in 1954. These lateral pterygoid muscular fibrous connections then form the interarticular disc in Meckel's cartilage by mechanical stimulation of this muscle[101]

Neurological, vascular, and ligamental communication between the TMJ and the middle ear is preserved during TMJ development and continues during adult life because of continuity of Meckel's cartilage through the petrotympanic fissure (causing an incomplete closing in adults). This fissure holds the chorda tympani nerve in its middle ear egress to the TMJ, amongst other ear-TMJ vestige structures. The medial pterygoid muscle and the tensor tympani muscle develop from the temporal blastema. These structures (along with the tensor veli palatine) are innervated by the trigeminal mandibular branch (V3), in turn innervating the masticatory muscles coming from the first branchial arch mesoderm.[102] Myrhaug[3] reasoned that the oscicular chain and middle ear muscles primarily belong to the chewing system (i.e. embryologically) but finally serve the auditory system.

The functional connection between the ear and TMJ in the adult arises from common phylogenetic establishment of both the ear and TMJ. Meckel's cartilage plays a role in organising and forming jointly-located anatomical structures (Figure 2).

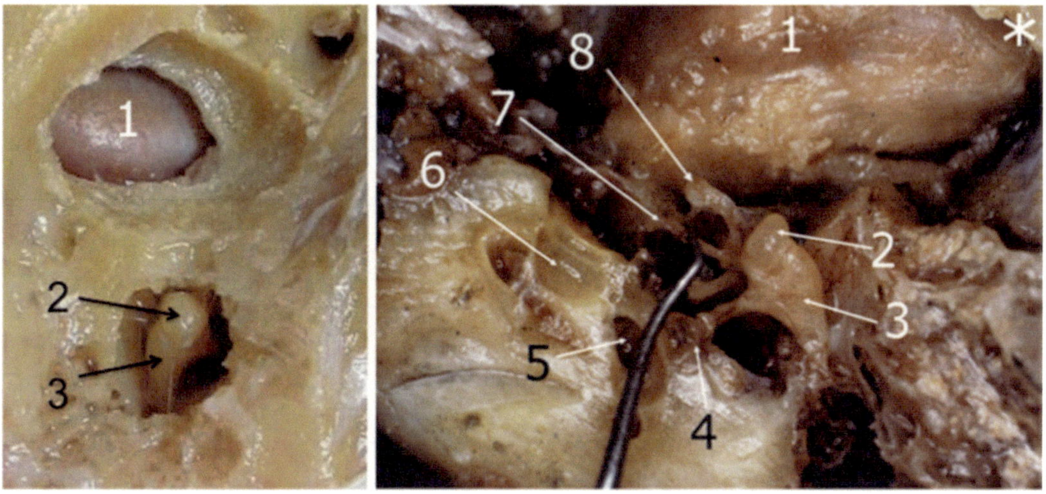

Fig. 2. TMJ and middle ear nearness in an temporal bone adult sample. 1. TMJ disc, 2. Malleus head, 3. Incus body, 4. Stape, 5. Inner ear vestibule, 6. Cochlea, 7. Chorda tympani nerve cut and medially pulled, 8. TMJ and malleus common ligaments cut. Author's dissection.

6. Muscular explanations

Complex neuromuscular interactions between masticatory muscles and ear muscles were called the "Otognatic Syndrome" by Myrhaug[3] and then the "Otomandibular Syndrome" by Arlen.[103] Otic symptoms in the otomandibular syndrome occur without a real source in the ear, nose, or throat but do involve one or more mastication muscles in a state of fatigue. Several interpretations exist involving multiple muscles.

6.1 First muscular exploration

Anatomically, the tensor tympani (malleus muscle; TT) and the tensor veli palatini (Eustachian tube muscle; TVP) are middle ear muscles; although, they are functionally modulated by trigeminal motor nucleus motoneurons, which also modulate six more mastication muscles larger in size. Although middle ear muscle function is far from being completely comprehended, it is possible that TT and TVP muscle participation in TMD may lead to otic referred consequences when there is a dysfunctional stomatognathic state.

The Eustachian tube connects the middle ear with the nasopharynx through the TVP, assisted by the levator palatini and salpingopharyngeus muscles during velopharyngeal movements such as swallowing and the inhaling phase of respiration, equalising external and internal pressures. Salen and Zakrisson[104] found that pharyngeal and laryngeal muscles simultaneously work with the TT during swallowing and assist in Eustachian tube ventilation in a similar way to that of an air pump. Normal movement patterns such as yawning, laughing, swallowing, and coughing involve pharyngeal and laryngeal muscles activating the TT and may contribute towards ventilating the middle ear. Table 2 shows common intratympanic and extratympanic movements for the TT, TVP, and stapedial muscles.

Muscles/ Movements	Tensor tympani Innervation: Trigeminal	Tensor veli palatini Innervation: Trigeminal	Stapedial Innervation: Facial
Speaking	X	X	
Chewing	X	X	
Swallowing	X	X	
Jawning	X	X	
Laughing	X	X	
Coughing	X	X	
Breathing	X	X	
Acoustic trauma	X		X
Before speaking	X		X
Palpebral reflex	X		X

Table 2. Common intratympanic and extratympanic movements.

Interestingly, otolaryngology and otology specialists have ignored the character of the TT function. Some physiologists attach to it the function of stretching the tympanic membrane for improved reception of sound energy, but in medical circles it is considered as a muscle with practically no function in sound transmission. In contrast, the stapedial muscle is recognized as a powerful muscle in sound modulation and auditory protection and there is also an awareness of how the paralysis of this muscle generates evident audiometric and clinical effects. It is also known that the stapedial muscle improves external vocalization, reducing the autogenous sound masking effect (auditory protective and discriminative function); however, the participation of the TT muscle in this remains unresolved.

Ramirez et al.[105] compared the length of the TT and stapedial muscles. The difference was a little more than three times greater between the length of the TT muscle and the stapedius muscle. During stapedial reflex there is a muscular movement of about 50 microns, which reduces sound transmission by approximately 50 dB bilaterally and improves perception by 50 dB. This forces us to reflect on the potential capacity of the TT in the medial mobilization of the tympanic membrane in protection and tuning mechanisms. It must be remembered that it measures three times more in length than the stapedius muscle and is connected to the oscicular chain through the malleus and almost in opposition vector to the stapedius muscle, which in theory could generate movements three times greater (approximately 150 microns) when activated. I wonder how a muscle of these dimensions can be considered as an unproductive muscle when it is known that the joint mechanics of the middle ear work with deformities around one nanometre, which explain the modulator power of the stapedial muscle. It must also be kept in mind that TT motor innervation depends entirely on the activation of the trigeminal motor nucleus, the almost exclusively neurological centre of the stomatognathic system.

TMD may produce constant (spastic) or episodic (clonic) contraction and tension in the TVP and TT muscles during a state of fatigue. Zipfel et al.[106] explained how in subjective tinnitus a "false sound perception" (only perceived by the person) have continuous or rhythmical contraction of the TT and stapedius muscles producing steady muscle contraction or myoclonus, which makes rhythmic movements on the stape annular membrane and in the tympanic membrane. Analogously, but excluding vascular abnormalities, a pulsate TVP muscle contraction during objective tinnitus, initiate a "true sound perception," (perceived by the operator too) with rhythmical opening and closing of the Eustachian tube's pharyngeal area (palatal myoclonus). An objective tinnitus can be produced by rhythmic movement during TT myoclonus or TVP myoclonus (Eustachian tube seal rhythmic opening 30 times per minute) in an individual or combined way. This involvement of these muscles can produce varying otic conductive behaviour, which may be tinnitus in fashioned forms.

6.2 Second muscular exploration

Oscicular chain equilibrium depends on the state of the opposing TT and stapedius muscle contraction (Figure 3), thus regulating the normal functioning of structures leading sound (acoustic compliance) into the middle ear.[107] Among incudo-malleolar and incudo-stapedial joints, it should be recognised that the oscicular chain in the middle ear is weakly supported by the tympanic membrane, some malleus and incus ligaments, the annular ligament, and stapedius and TT muscle tendons. These structures support middle ear bones in a delicate but biomechanically efficient arrangement for receiving and transmitting acoustic stimuli to the inner ear. Although differently innervated (VII pair), the stapedius muscles accompany

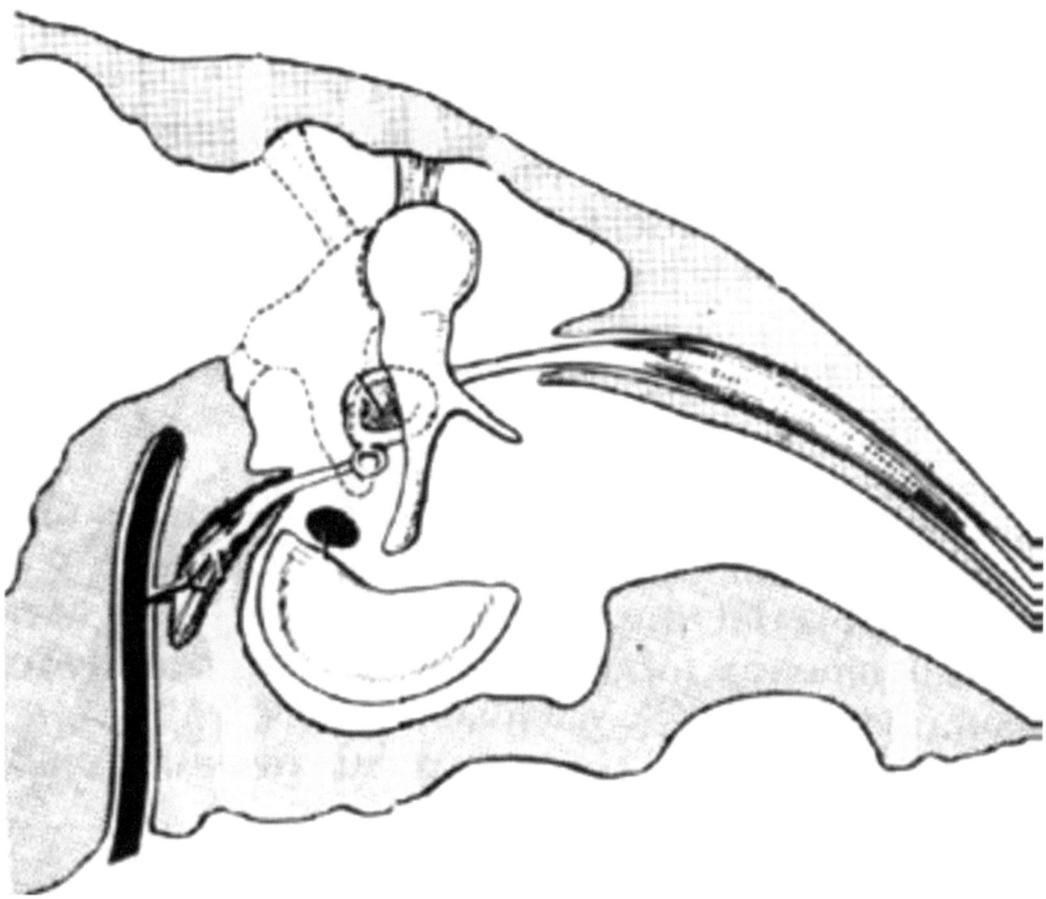

Fig. 3. Tensor tympani and stapedial muscles in the middle ear cavity. Modification from Bouchet & Guilleret´s Anatomy. Ed. Panamericana.

the TT muscle in auditory conduction during middle ear protection and filtering mechanisms, due to tympanic membrane stiffness regulation (Figure 4). Stapedius and TT muscle contraction is produced during many normal events. Also, they can be stimulated by the CNS in centrifuge auditory inhibition control (olivocochlear efferent system), protecting and filtering auditory afferent conduction towards the CNS through contracting these muscles and by additional inner ear hair cell modification.[108] Such combined stapedial and TT muscle mechanisms normally work by discriminating, fine-tuning, and improving external vocalisation; reducing the masking effect of autogenous sounds (pre-vocalisation contraction); enhancing transient stimuli against continuous background noise; and responding to strong external stimuli, protecting against possible acoustic trauma. It may be activated by vocalisation, chewing, swallowing, and facial muscle movement.[109]

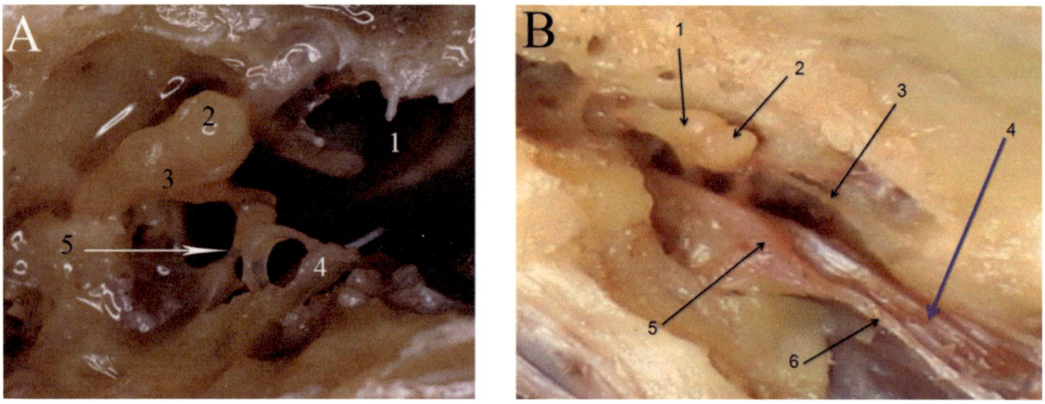

Fig. 4. Human temporal specimen's middle ear and middle cranial fossae. A: 1. Tympanic membrane, 2. Malleus head, 3. Incus, 4. Stape, 5. (Arrow) Stapedial muscle´s tendon emerging from Pyramidal aphophysis. B: 1. Incus, 2. Malleus head, 3. Chorda tympani nerve, 4. Tensor tympani muscle, 5. Geniculate ganglion, 6. Superficial petrosal nerve. Author's dissection.

TT muscle has a high threshold (100 dB), a latency of 12 ms and large and variable amplitude, which can be masked by stapedial muscle during impedance test, due to their lower threshold (70 dB) and latency (7 ms). Through electromyography and genetic testing in other species TT muscle (as stapedial muscle) has been shown to has special contractile properties and resistant to fatigue because of its fast oxidative glycolytic fibers.[110] The mechanical application of acoustic stimuli (70-100 dB frequency of 2 KHz) is responded immediately due to this feature.[111] According to Ochi et al.[112], the activity of the TT muscle (in addition to the centrifuge auditory inhibition control originated in the cochlea) can be evoked from somato-sensory or sensori-vestibular origins. With this in mind, a complex physiological activity of TT muscle cannot be forgotten, especially when hearing, protecting, discriminating, autogenous sound-enmascaring and pressure equalizing multiple functions offers a paramount role in middle ear.

In 1987, Malkin[113] stated that the TT serves as a barometric pressure receiver. Its propioceptive afference signals (starting from their muscular length) can be triggered in a hypotonic situation caused by low tympanic cavity pressure (due to mucosal air exchange). Such low-pressure medially retracts the tympanic membrane and TT tendon due to great external environmental pressure accompanied by no resistance to force; its muscular spindles perceive such new muscle elongation. The trigeminal motor nucleus produces a reflex mechanism in a polysynaptic central arrangement, beginning TT muscle contraction involving opening the Eustachian tube (through TVP activation), middle ear ventilation and pressure equilibration; such normal physiological mechanisms may be blocked by the TT fatigued and hypertonic scenario during TMD.

Klockhoff and Anderson[114] proposed a "TT syndrome" when the above cannot function correctly during TMD. Sustained TT muscle contraction during TMD can alter the oscicular spatial position and perilymphatic and endolymphatic pressure through the transmitted changes from the oval window to the cochlea and semicircular canal walls. It should be stressed that the auditive cells are very sensitive and constantly depolarise even during rest (spontaneous otoacoustic emissions), which may be perceived as tinnitus by some patients. Sensorial spontaneous otoacoustic emissions can be mechanically increased (conductively) by the TT and stapedius spasm, or myoclonus. Moreover, the TMD pathogenic scenario regarding middle ear muscle mechanisms may abnormally reduce sonic transmitting vibration from the tympanic membrane towards the oval window, which may be expressed as a paroxistic subjective hearing loss. This anomalous muscular-oscicular relationship may also trigger abnormal mechanical sensory organ stimuli and unbalance vestibular impulses. This entire situation may be expressed as tinnitus, subjective hearing loss, and vertigo.[115]

6.3 Third muscular exploration

The shortening and thickening of the mastication medial pterygoid muscle in over-closed jaw positions (specially in edentulous patients) can produce an anatomical cross-sectional widening area that exerts a lateral pulling force on the adjacent TVP muscle and the Eustachian tube (Figure 5).[116] Mistaken vertical dimension rehabilitation is common in edentulous patients with a varied referred symptoms presentation caused by this clinical situation (Figure 6). Goto et al,[117] explained that an increase of medial pterygoid transverse volume can result from an open-closed position depending on muscle length and tension variation. The close proximity of both muscles can normally be observed during TVP muscle

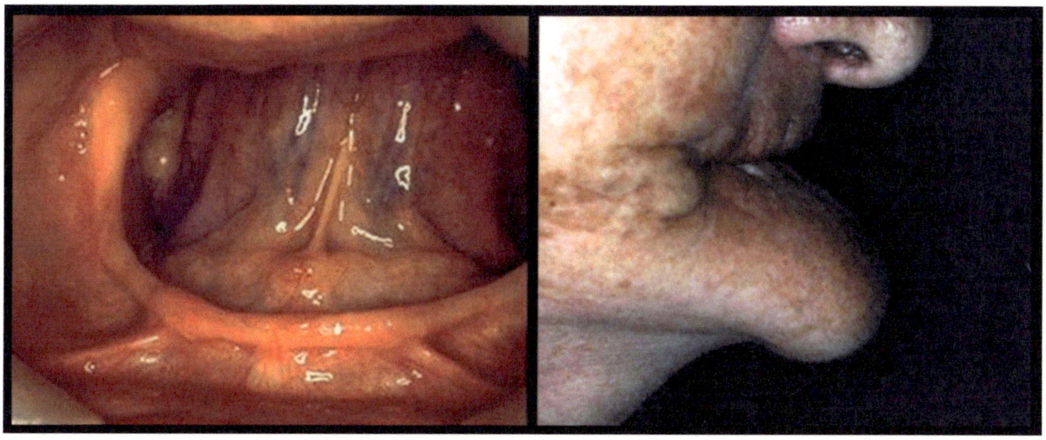

Fig. 5. Intraoral and extraoral view of edentulous patient with referred otic symptoms originated in an advanced jaw osseous reabsorption with overclosure prosthesis (not showed) that do not regain a normal intermaxilar vertical dimension. Photography use authorized to the author (Patient's record).

contraction, which opens the Eustachian tube lumen and laterally presses on the medial pterygoid muscle (Figure 7). Sehhati-Chafai-Leuwer et al.[118] named this contact "hypomochlia," or fulcrum, stating that it can change muscle tension direction together with another two structures contacting the TVP (pterygoid hamulus and Ostmann's fatty tissue), which may influence middle ear ventilation by Eustachian tube compliance.

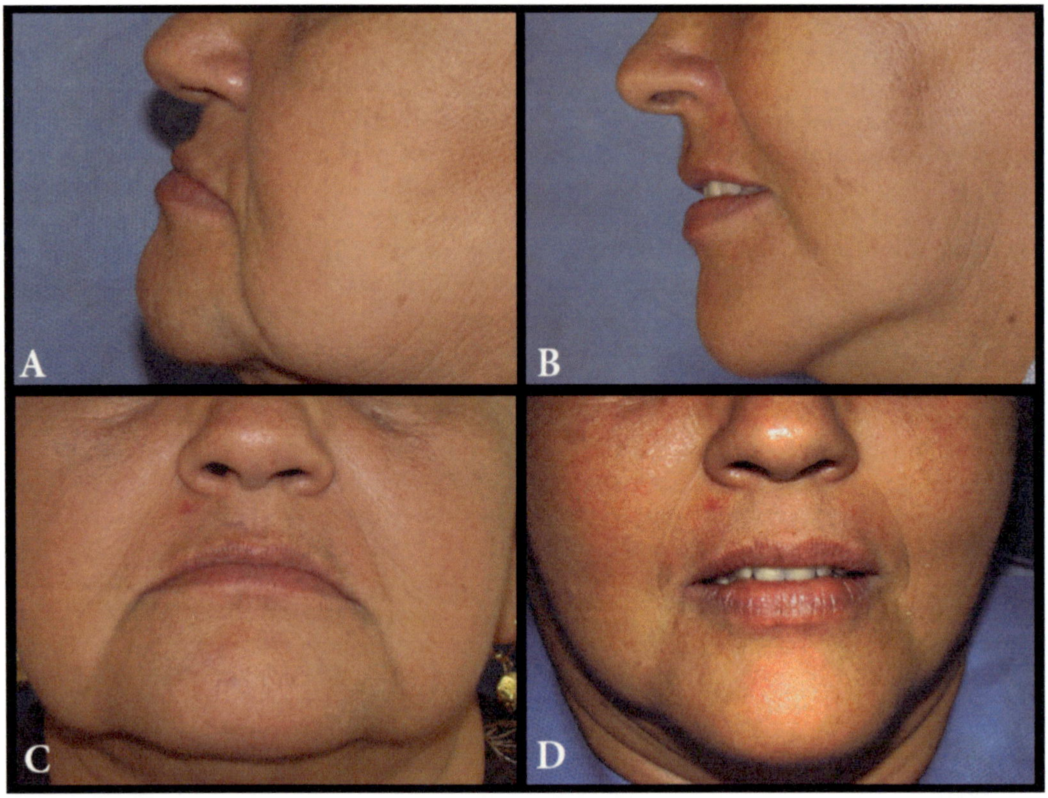

Fig. 6. Frontal and lateral photographic registration with an incorrect (A,C) and a correct complete denture vertical dimension rehabilitation. Photography use authorized to the author (Patient's record).

A deep overbite, medial pterygoid shortening, hypertonicity, or spasm results in muscular mass compression and lateral bunching of the adjacent TVP and associated structures.[119,120] If masticatory muscles are hypertonic because of a TMD, the TVP and TT muscles may be hypertonic due to equal innervation by V3. Penkner et al.[121] stated the opposite in a pilot-study with 16 TMD patients tested with an EMG needle and audio and tympanogram recordings, which did not provide a correlation with such dysfunction. However, in the Penkner et al. study, the patient population was small and their research design lacked a control group; moreover, it did not have an evident chronic TMD group or a satisfactory group with severe dysfunction (only two patients). Dysfunctional TVP was not present in that study, because all patients demonstrated regular and bilateral opening of the Eustachian tube.

It must be considered that the TVP and TT have gained embryological, anatomical, physiological, and neurological territory in the stomatognathic system, and research regarding them is complex and sensitive (requiring precision). A good methodological design could

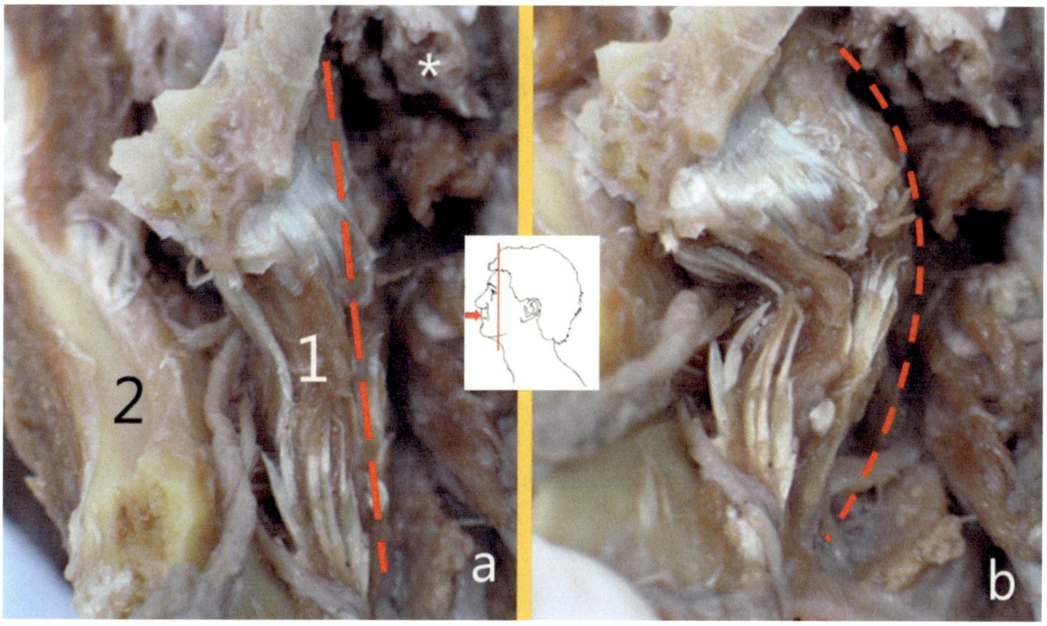

Fig. 7. Jaw and pharyngeal area frontal view: Medial Pterygoid and Eustaquian tube dissection. Picture a- Jaw in normal vertical dimension: 1. Medial pterygoid muscle, 2. Sectioned frontal jaw body, *. Eustaquian tube cartilage. Picture b- Jaw in overclosure position increasing medial pterygoid transverse volume on Eustaquian tube cartilague. Author's dissections.

discard or confirm a probable cause-effect relationship between Eustachian tube dysfunction and TVP dysfunction.

McDonnell et al.[122] stated that children with deep dental overbites were 2.8 times more likely to develop Eustachian tube dysfunction than those without deep overbites because of the muscular over-closed position. Azadani et al.[123] affirm that children with deep bites were 10.6 times more prone to Eustachian tube dysfunction than those without deep bites in their multivariate model.

Interestingly, although infection is the most prevalent aetiology of otitis media in children (allergic conditions or respiratory infections), TVP dysfunction (TMD) may also produce otitis media with effusion.[124] It is well known that the middle ear transudation effect is due to hypoventilation and abnormal gas exchange when the Eustachian tube becomes blocked and impeded to regulate pressure. The Eustachian tube normally maintains a closed position at rest, protecting the middle ear from retrograde nasopharynx microflora flow during rapid fluctuations in nasopharyngeal pressure associated with breathing, swallowing, coughing, sneezing, and nose-blowing. Children's Eustachian tube dysfunction plays an important role because of the anatomical configuration of the Eustachian tube (short, horizontal, and wide lumen) or the TVP open-closed dynamics is spastic or trapped by the neighbouring pterygoid muscle.[125]

6.4 Fourth muscular exploration

It is reasonable to propose that if TT and TVP dysfunction can separately produce otic symptoms, then the effects of an anatomically agonistic co-working function may be more problematic. Barsoumian et al.[126] corroborated Lupin's 1969 findings and Rood and Doyle's[127] results by discovering how the fibres of the most external TVP muscle area and the TT fibres are joined in the middle ear in adult human cadavers (Figure 8).[128] The TVP thus has an additional bone origin in the malleus manubrium. Kierner et al.[129] corroborated this functional connection in human cadavers through histological analysis. TT and TVP dysfunction in TMD can modify the malleus and tympanic membrane's medial position, individually or in combination (inner deflection). Consequently, these muscles act synergistically together and can temporarily increase a medial intra-tympanic pulling force effect with the expected otic referred symptom consequence, due to such delicate oscicular chain biomechanics. A macroscopically morphological study found these same connection fibers between TT and TVP muscles in 23 human temporal blocks (Figure 9 and 10).[5] This proves the anterior histological and anatomical findings about the possible combined function between TVP and TT muscles with its masticatory-otic dysfunctional referred symptoms consequences. After all, understanding middle ear ventilation physiology through the Eustachian tube involves neurological territories referred from the stomatognathic system that considers TT and TVP muscle vital.

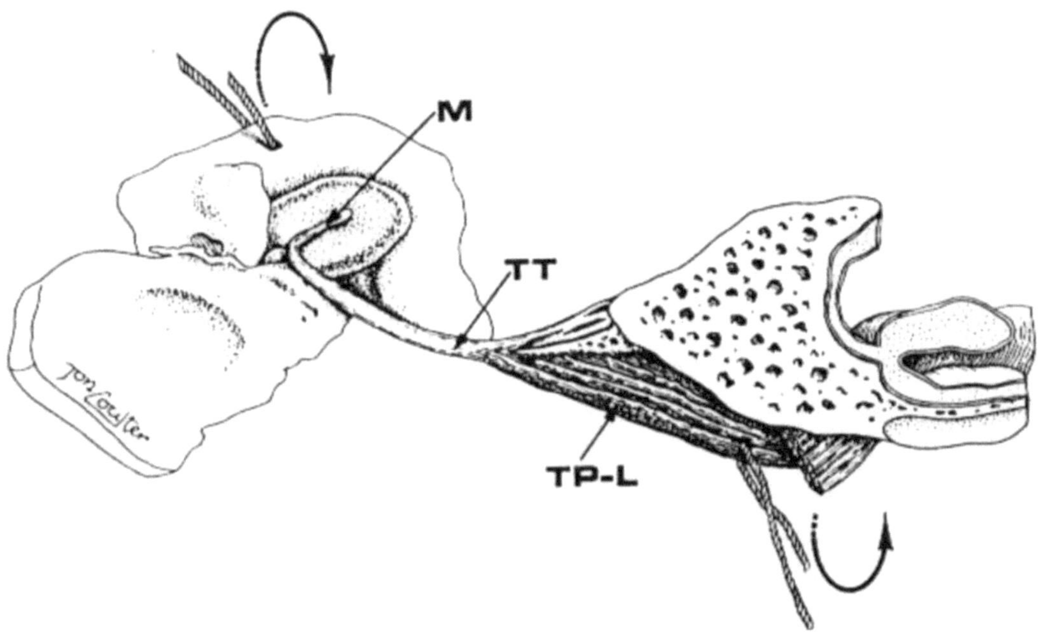

Fig. 8. TT and TVP muscle fiber connection. M. Malleus manubrium, TT. Tensor tympani muscle, TP-L. Tensor veli palatini muscle. Used with author´s permission from Rood, S.R. & Doyle, W.J. (1978). Morphology of tensor veli palatini, tensor tympani, and dilatator tubae muscles. Ann Otol Rhinol Laryngol, 87:202-10.

6.5 Fifth muscular exploration

Several studies have investigated concomitant functional connections between TMD and cervical spine disorders.[130,131] The functionality of cervical and masticatory systems is complemented synergistically but pathologically too in a concomitant way. Kuttila et al.[75] reported that 45% of TMD-tinnitus patients have headaches and 54% have neck-shoulder

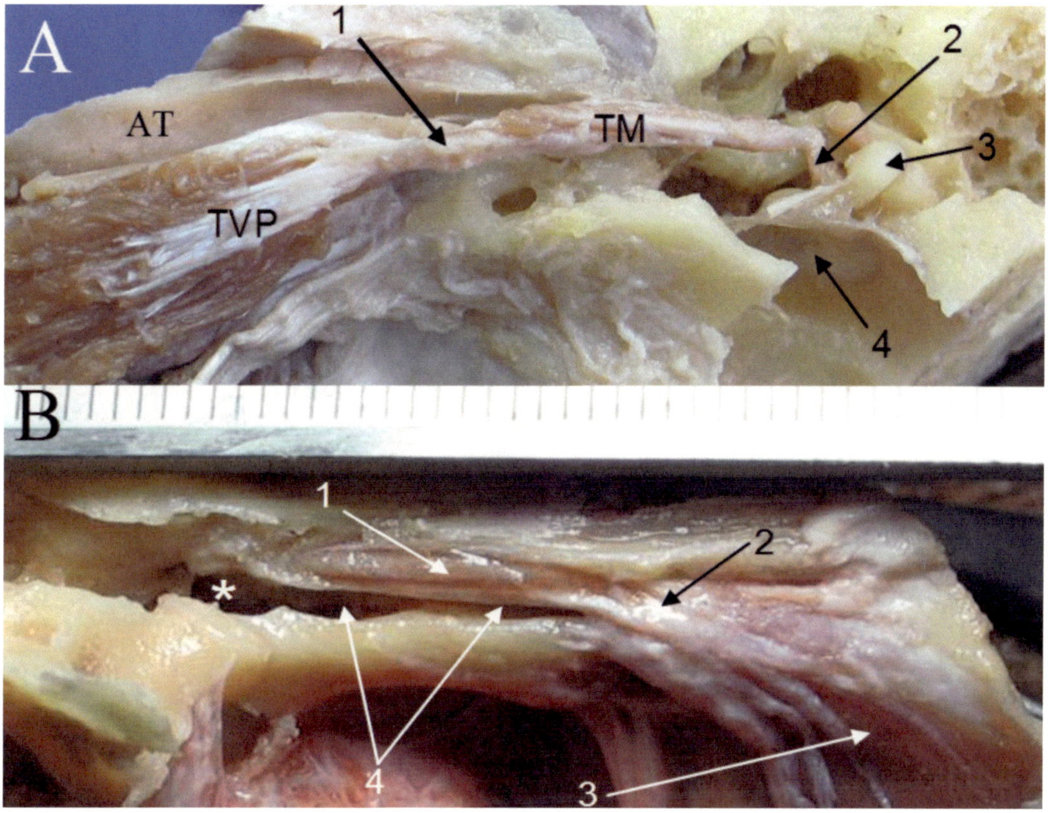

Fig. 9. Dissections on TT and TVP muscle fiber connections. A: AT, Auditory tube, TVP. Tensor veli palatine muscle, TM, Tensor tympani muscle, 1. Fiber connection, 2. Tensor tympani muscle´s tendon, 3. Malleus head, 4. Tympanic membrane. B: 1. Tenor tympani muscle, 2. Fiber connection, 3. Tensor veli palatine muscle, 4. Osseous portion of Eustaquian´s tube, *. Tympanic cavity. Author's dissections.

pain. Levine et al.[78] were able to produce cranio-cervical tinnitus modulation in normal otologic patients (tinnitus and non-tinnitus patients) using isometric cephalo-cervical exercises changing the loudness, pitch, and location of tinnitus by modulating the somatosensory and acoustic central neural pathway. If cranial and cervical muscular dysfunction in TMD (producing hypertonicity and muscular spasm) can trigger tinnitus, then it can also irritate nerves and blood vessels by muscular trapping. Cervical muscular fatigue may produce tension on the vertebral artery which feeds the basilar artery and inner ear inflow, with exacerbated otic consequences.[78,79] Additionally, it may also distort normal propioceptive reception in the vestibular nucleus and in the cervico-oculo-vestibular muscle reflex controlling the head's postural position, thereby complicating neck-otic vascular flow and worsening the vertigo produced.

7. Temporal bone explanations

TMJ and middle ear have a bone communication (iter chorda anterious) known as Huguier's channel that is shown by dry and fresh dissections in Figure 11 and 12. The TMJ and middle

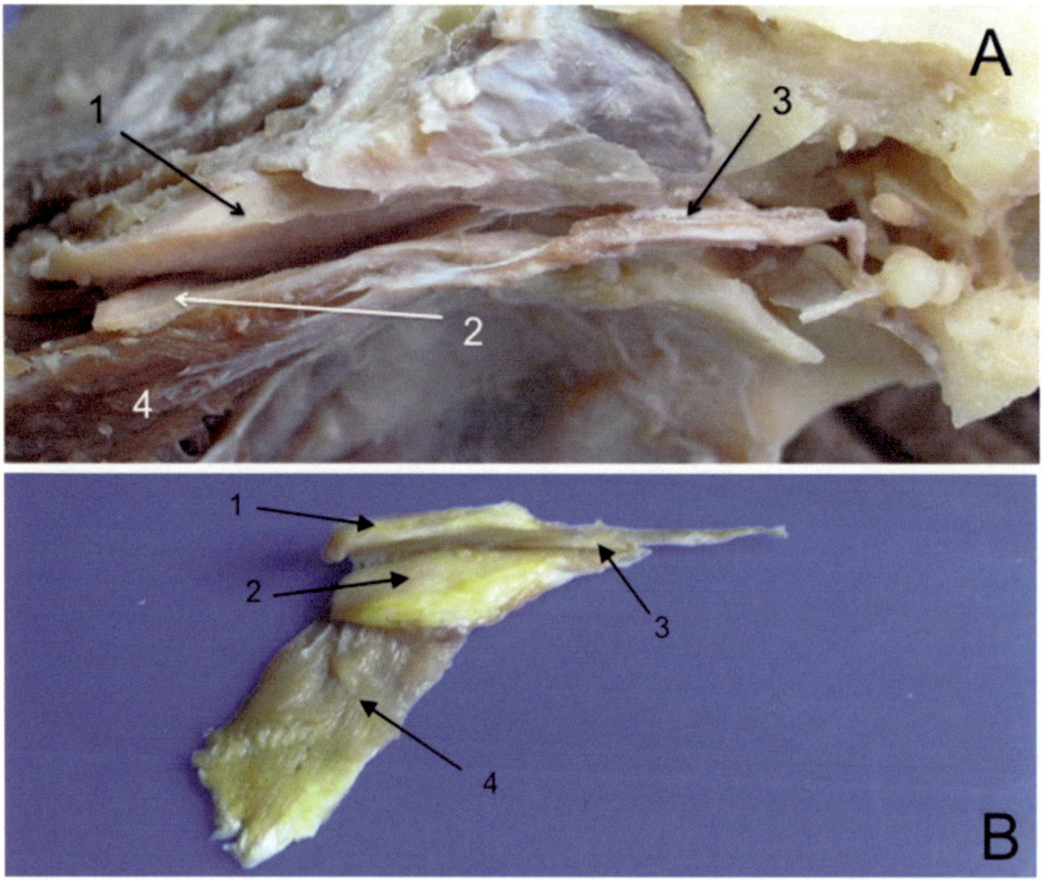

Fig. 10. Dissections on TT and TVP muscles related to left cartilaginous and mucous Eustaquian tube. A: Structure in situ. B: Structure block retired from temporal bone. 1 and 2. Hemisected Eustaquian tube. 3. Tenor tympani muscle, 4. Tensor veli palatine muscle, Author's dissections.

ear are small, compact structures that share through this communication vascular (anterior tympanic and deep auricular arteries), neurological (chorda tympani and auriculotemporal nerve), and ligamental: disco-malleolar ligament (DML) and anterior malleolar ligament (AML). These can be easily injured during TMJ disorder and may explain associated otic symptoms.[132,133]

7.1 First bone common passages exploration:

Human adult and foetus dissection has confirmed an anatomical link between the TMJ, the mandibular body, and the middle ear.[134,135,136,137,138,139,140141,142,143,144] DML and AML are responsible for such bone communication and connection; they are attached to the oscicular chain (malleus) and may create a biomechanical connection between the middle ear and the mandible.[145,146,147,148] These findings is corroborated in 23 human temporal bone specimens (Figure 13) that consistently show these ligamental structures.[149]

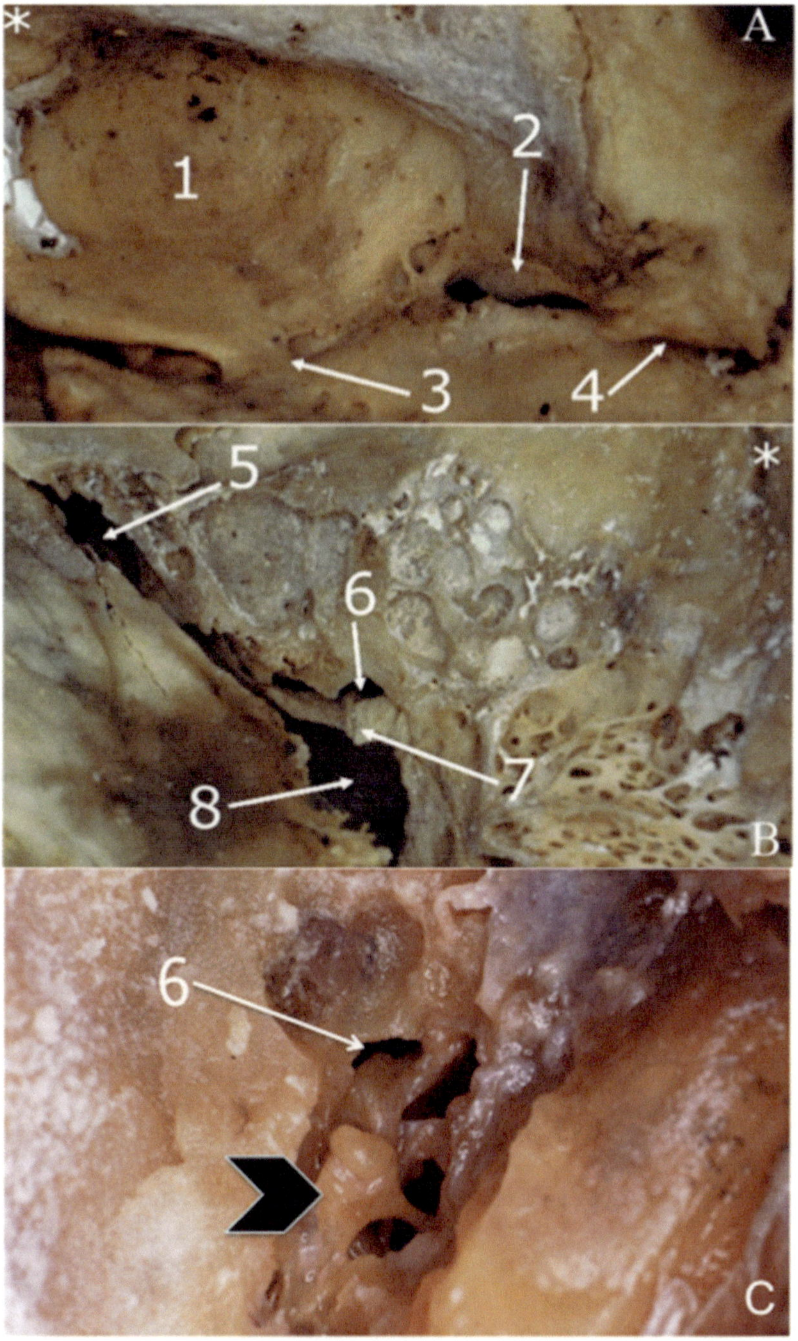

Fig. 11. A. External view of Huguier's canal from TMJ. B. Internal view of Huguier's canal from middle ear. * Antero-lateral sample orientation. C. Internal fresh view with ossicular chain (Arrow head). 1. TMJ fossae, 2. Huguier's canal external foramen, 3. Scamo-tympanic fissure, 4. Petro-tympanic fissure, 5. Auditive tube osseous portion, 6. Huguier's canal internal foramen, 7. Huguier's canal septum, 8. Tympanic cavity. Author's dissections.

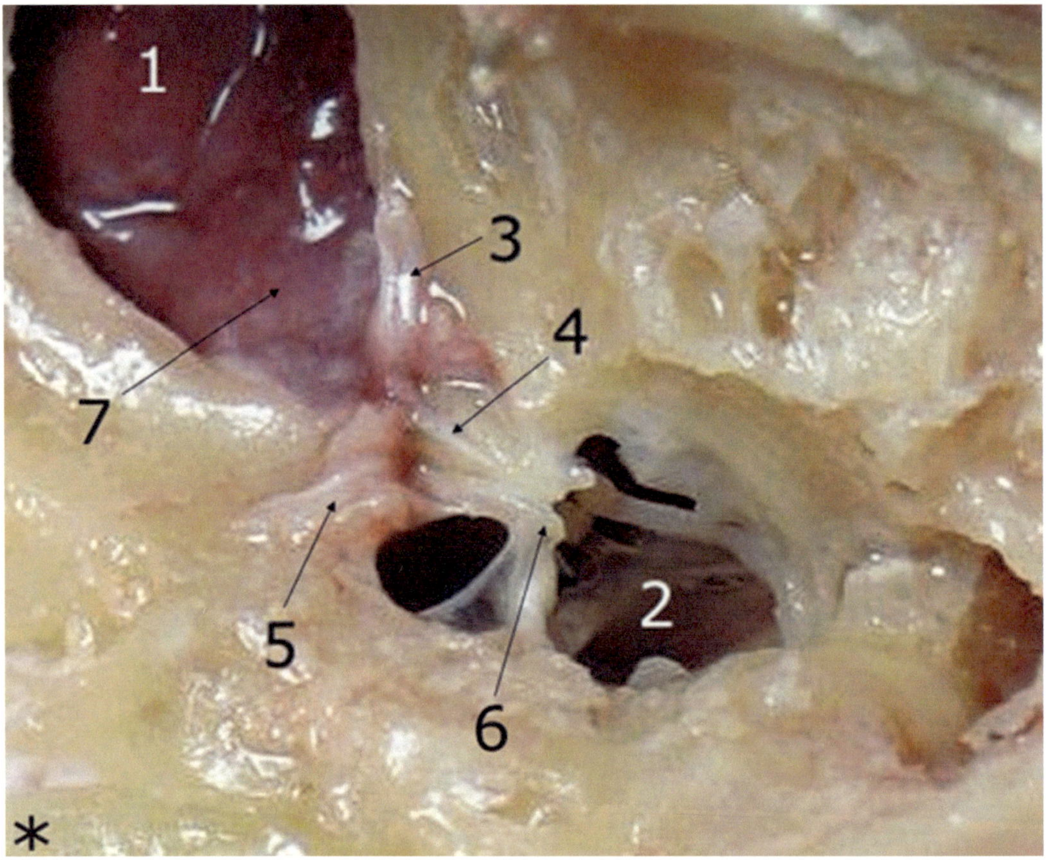

Fig. 12. Superior and postero-medial view of right middle ear and TMJ. * Postero-medial sample orientation. 1. TMJ disc, 2. Middle ear, 3. DML antero-laterally separated from the lateral side of Huguier's canal, 4. DML and AML Huguier's canal septum, 5. AML antero-medially separated from the medial side of Huguier's canal, 6. Chorda tympani nerve supraseptal trajectory, 7. TMJ bilaminar zone. Author's dissections.

These ligamental structures may be stretched by a TMJ disorder, which could affect middle ear oscicular equilibrium; although, there is controversy about their ability to disturb the oscicular chain.[150,151,152,153] The spread of forces through cranial bone sutures was treated by Libin in 1987 and suggested that ligaments common to neighbouring structures could become tensioned during normal physiological mobilization and in abnormal temporal bone trauma.[154] Retrodiscal tissue elasticity can normally act as an energy buffer in spreading movement from the TMJ to the middle ear by such common ligaments; however, TMJ disc luxation or oedematous pressure from an inflammatory disorder could certainly cause tension on the malleus through Huguier's canal.[133,155,156]

The range of tympanic membrane deformation during conducting sound energy must be understood when trying to ascertain the possibility of motion from the DML and AML on malleus oscicles. Tonndorf et al.[157] used time-average holography to show that an intense acoustic stimulus (111-121 dB) can deform the tympanic membrane by no more than nanometers or possibly a micrometer, depending on the frequency and place for tympanic

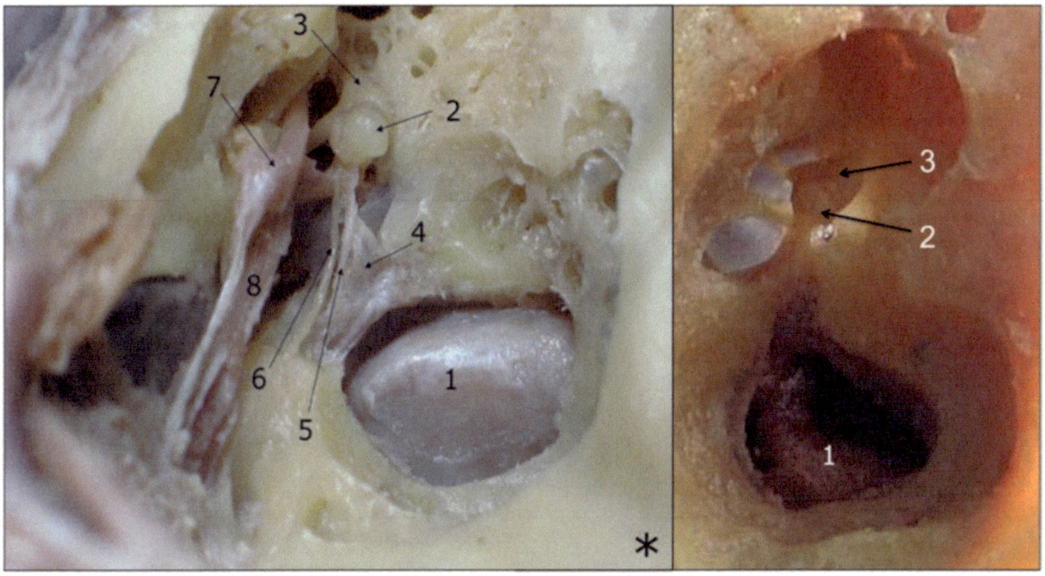

Fig. 13. Superior and antero-medial view of left middle ear and TMJ. * Antero-lateral sample orientation. 1. TMJ disc, 2. Malleus head, 3. Incus, 4. DML, 5. AML, 6. Chorda tympani nerve, 7. VII cranial pair geniculated ganglion, 8. tensor tympani muscle. Author's dissections.

membrane measurement.[158] Tympanic membrane and middle ear vibration produced by sound energy is thus on the nanometer range scale. The auditory threshold thus responds from sub-angstrom oscicular motion.[159,160] This finding has been widely corroborated by Wada et al.[161,162] using better-quality tympanometry equipment with low probe tone frequency (time-average speckle pattern interferometry) and finite element analysis at different frequencies and pressures in human and other species' hearing systems.

According to Eckerdal[150], the range of movement of these ligaments depends on the fibrous connection on the walls of the petrotympanic fissure, thereby corroborating Coleman's findings[138]. Ramirez et al.,[149] findings concern 30.5% DML's malleolar mobility correlated well with Sato et al.[163] who showed a spacious Huguier's canal in 29.2% of samples, suggesting a wide foramen which could allow free passage of its inner structures. If the oscicular chain can transmit a nonometric tympanic vibration through two joints (from tympanic membrane to inner ear), with more than four ligaments and two muscles having an effective area and lever relationship, it would thus be potential that DML and AML have a highly probable movement effect on oscicular chain spatial disposition when TMJ-jaw traction is applied to them by the malleus.

Experiments have demonstrated that AML fixation (producing stiffness) is dominant at low frequencies. Although low frequency tinnitus has been reported to be very rare and diverse (it may vary in pitch from low to high frequency, intermittent or permanent and vary in intensity), it cannot be ruled out that it is caused by oscicular fixation and/or a low admittance pattern. The work of Nakajima et al.[164] has ruled out the idea that ligamental motion may not produce an auditory effect by appreciable excitation of the inner ear due to high-pass filtering by different systems (helicotrema, incudo-malleolar, incudo-stapedial and oval anullar ligament joints). They revealed reduced auditory sensitivity (8-10 dB loss) when the AML was partially fixed and a larger loss (15-35 dB) when it was totally fixed. This proved that restraining the oscicles produced an increase in the ear's impedance. They tried to simulate an otosclerosis lesion because AML fixation clinically occurs in combination with this pathology.[165] This experimental model also proved the power of adjustment in sound transmission of this ligament.[166] In this sense, whether such motion at low frequencies involved in TMJ-jaw motion can produce enough sound to be heard at an auditory threshold close to 1 Hz (the stapes move at least one micron) is not suspicious.

Huguier's canal's morphological dimensions play a paramount role in the above possibility. Huguier's canal has a slender funnel-like form in the petrotympanic fissure (being wider near the TMJ and narrower near the middle ear). Sato et al.[163] and Eckerdal[150] measured such dimensions at three sagittal places (near the TMJ, the middle area and near the middle ear) agreeing a plentiful wide space dimensions. Such Huguier's canal morphology suggests permissive movement ability for the DML and AML when a force is applied to them and transmitted via oscicular chain vibration dynamics. In a partial agreement with Eckerdal[150] (Huguier's canal adherence restricting ligaments mobility), I do not consider such adherence able to impede nanometer movement transmission in a collagenous (and maybe elastic) ligament from TMJ anterior traction force during protrusion. Riga et al.,[62] demonstrated an increase in stiffness of the middle ear of forty patients with TMD that could demonstrate minor conductive alterations of the middle ear by these mechanisms that generate referred otic symptoms from TMJ.

Differing explanations have arisen from these ligaments' morphology regarding Huguier's canal dimensions, strengthened by oscicular chain dynamics' physiology. Cheng[167] found AML good viscoelastic performance calculated for tension resistance (1.05 MPa) and stretching resistance (1.51 MPa), thereby assuring force transmission from the TMJ to the middle ear malleus. Disorganized surface collagen disposition was found regarding this structure's morphology (trespassing Huguier's canal walls), enveloping a wide and well-organized internal longitudinal collagen band ordered as a double collagen layer assembly with a thin disorganized external stratum. This characteristic, plus its width, mechanical resistance and sound energy transmission magnitude, makes Eckerdal's adherence model for Huguier's canal doubtful.

Normal excursion of the disc and condyle during mandibular movement (Figure 14) may not provoke malleus mobility and altered tympanic membrane tension; however, functional or inflammatory joint disorders such as disc luxation or secondary oedema may produce oscicular chain tension by disco-malleolar ligament traction.[155,156,168] Ren et al.,[169] found a significant correlation between internal TMJ derangement and tinnitus, detecting disk luxation in the ipsilateral joint of 53 patients with unilateral tinnitus.[170] Kuttila et al.[75] found a similar relationship between TMJ internal derangement and tinnitus. According to this hypothesis, tinnitus and vertigo may originate in the altered stapes' position due to the force being transmitted from these malleus ligaments. Likewise, otalgia may be present because of peripheral nerve stimulation in the tympanic membrane due to membrane-bonded malleus traction.

In relation to the spheno-mandibular ligament, there is agree with the findings of Abe et al.,[171] who found that this ligament was inferiorly fixed to the mandible and superiorly fixed to the sphenoid spine and the anterior malleolar ligament as shown by personal dissections on human temporal bone specimens (Figure 15). Both may be tensed in a marked over-closure position, also stretching oscicular balance. The otic effects are latent in this tensed

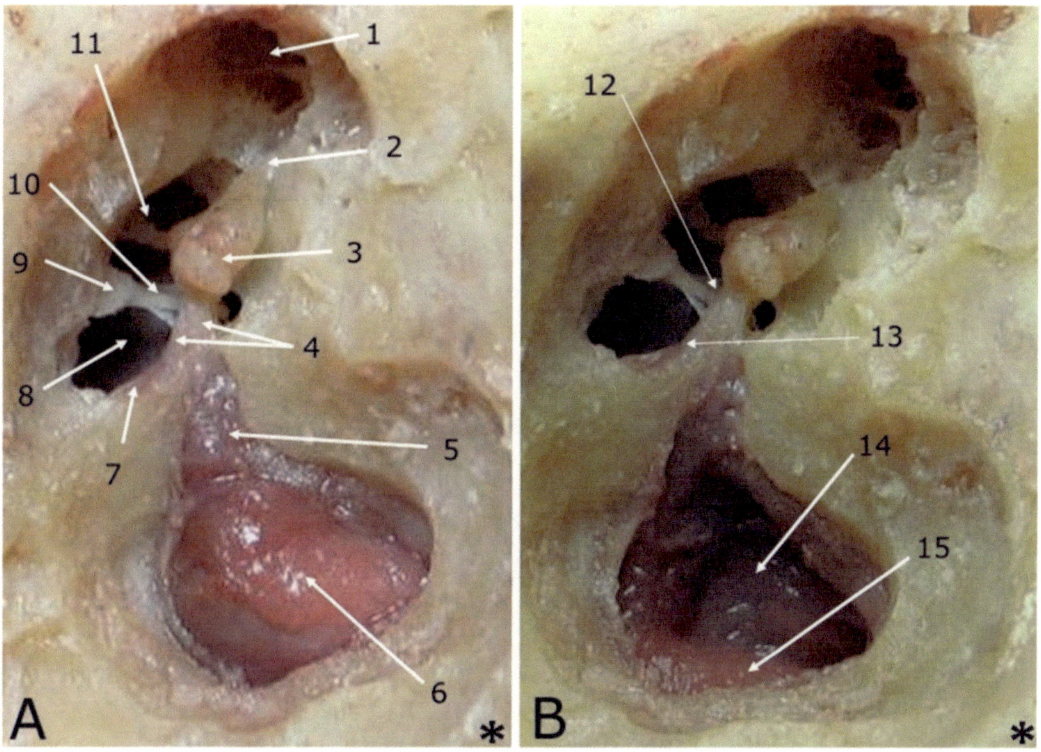

Fig. 14. Superior and antero-medial view of left middle ear and the TMJ. TMJ's disc anterior traction protrusion). * Antero-lateral sample orientation. Fig. A, 1. Mastoid aditus, 2. Incudal fossa, 3. incudo-malleolar joint, 4. DML (short arrow) and AML (long arrow) emerging from the malleus anterior process, 5. DML fixing to TMJ bilaminar zone, 6. TMJ disc, 7. AML in its supra-septal medial course, 8. Internal face of tympanic membrane, 9. Chocleariform process, 10. Tensor tympani muscle tendon, 11. Incudo-stapedial joint, 12. Chorda tympani nerve over tensor tympani muscle tendon, 13. Chorda tympani nerve and AML medial course, 14. TMJ bilaminar zone stretched in excursive tractional TMJ movements, 15. TMJ disc in extreme protrusive movement. Author's dissections.

mechanical scenario, especially in edentulous patients. Alkofide et al.,[146] studied anterior malleolar and spheno-mandibular ligaments structural characteristics in 37 specimens, determining that the spheno-mandibular one reached the malleus (8.1%) and the middle ear (67.6%), whilst the anterior malleolar one passed through the petrotympanic fissure with the spheno-mandibular (58.3%), suggesting guaranteed connectivity between both ligaments. Burch[145] found that spheno-mandibular ligament relaxed during maximum jaw opening and tensed during over closure; however, it has been suggested that it can be stretched during lateral jaw movements too.[172] Both ligaments can thus be tensioned in several situations, which may alter the oscicular chain,[173] although I could not observe this in my dissections.

7.2 Second bone common passages exploration

The vascular relationship between the TMJ and the middle ear may explain otic symptoms in the presence of a vascular reflex from TMJ disorders. The most medial anterior tympanic artery posterior group branches (behind the TMJ) irrigate the tympanic cavity and the

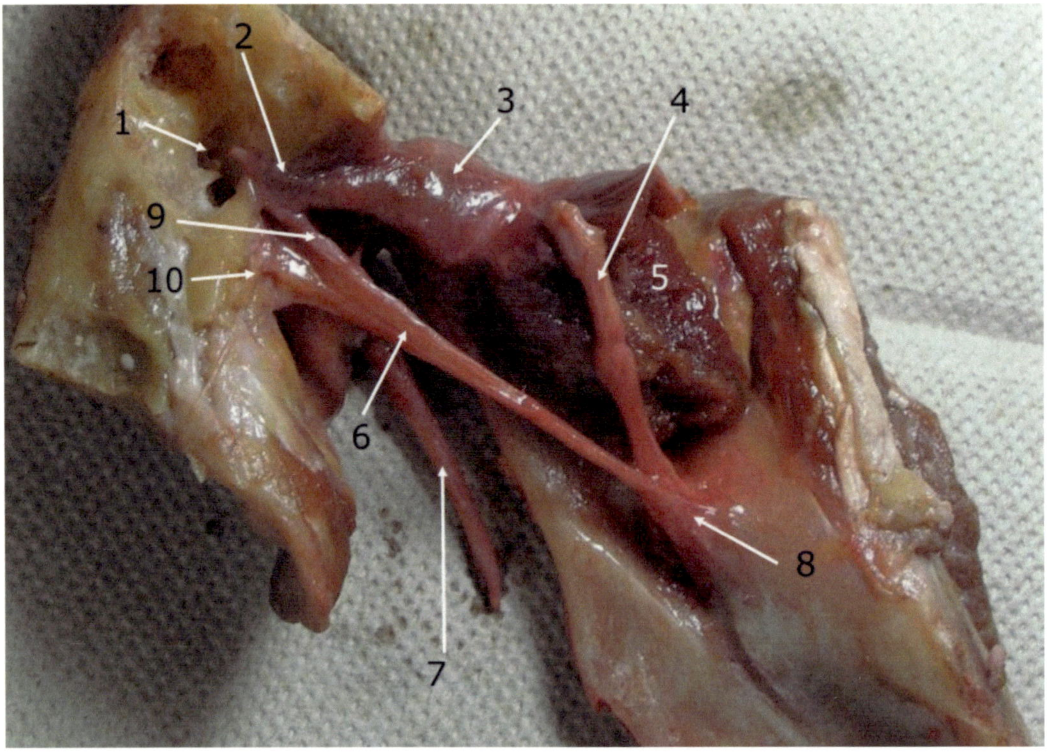

Fig. 15. Left TMJ, mandible ramus and middle ear medial view. 1. Tympanic cavity, 2. DML bilaminar area union, 3. TMJ disc, 4. Alveolar nerve sectioned and retracted over external pterygoid muscle, 5. External pterygoid muscle, 6. EML, 7. Styloid process, 8. Lingula, 9. AML fixing to EML lateral surface, 10. Sphenoid spine. Author's dissections.

external auditory meatus through the petrotympanic fissure, using the same osseous routes as the ligaments, as explained above[141]. Moreover, Merida-Velasco et al.[174] found how the small venous vessels from the anterior portion of the middle ear (crossing the petrotympanic fissure) reach the venous retrodiscal plexus and drain into the retromandibular vein. Interrupting normal artery flow may affect the auditory system.

7.3 Third bone communication exploration

Marasa and Ham[125] suggested that oedema produced by TMJ inflammatory disorders could spread through the petrotympanic fissure to the middle ear and produce serous otitis media. Oedema produced in the TMJ can spread collected fluid through the petrotympanic fissure to the middle ear and produce vulnerable disease via this route.[175] Osseous communication between the middle ear and TMJ in children may lead to pathologies such as TMJ septic arthritis (with a doubtful infectious site), in the presence of infectious otitis media.[176,177]

8. Is TMD integrated in an otic multidimensional model?

The question is still open regarding the hierarchy of peripheral and/or central sources of otic symptoms and how they appear to interact in a simultaneous way. Rubinstein et al.,[178] reported that TMD patients with a longer duration of tinnitus responded worse to the TMD treatment than those with a shorter duration, suggesting peripheral acute pathology and central neuroplastic change during chronic symptoms, implying a combination of them. This dichotomy is well pictured in Abel at al.,[79] works on somatomotor-somatosensorial tinnitus modulation.[78] However, these modulations were only recognised as otic sensori-neuronal phenomenon, without allowing for an otic conductive scenario. Jaw movement needs trigeminal motor nucleus motoneuron intervention activating the TT and TVP with expected conductive effects.

It is difficult to take a solely neuroanatomical or neurophysiologic viewpoint when interpreting otic symptoms due to combined peripheral-central interactions, particularly in the absence of objective and unique neurological signs and intricate auditory and stomatognathic system connections at different CNS levels. Interspecies and human neuroanatomy provide the most important advances on the influence of some tracts and cortical areas on others and how they may be felt as secondary sensorineural otic symptoms. The protagonism of constant deep pain, trigemino-vascular auditive control, somatosensorial-auditory multimodal integration, cortical and subcortical sound broadband interpretation, corticofugal modulation, and limbic behavioural interferences as CNS phenomena has been demonstrated in referred otic symptom pathophysiology. However, CNS dynamics-initiated associated symptoms also have a relevant peripheral feedback effect on auditory cortical and subcortical connections that can be additionally produced and modified by a conductive intermediate level (middle ear).

9. Evidence regarding dental treatment outcome

There are many forms of otic treatment, such as pharmacological, surgical, instrumental, phychophysiological, counselling, electrostimulatory, physiotherapy (cervical spine mobility), acupuncture, hypnosis, thermotherapy, cryotherapy, ultrasound-laser therapy, biofeedback, and stomatognathic treatment[68]. Stomatognathic treatment addressing masticatory muscle relaxation (including the TT and TVP) by using removable interocclusal plastic appliances seems to be able to eliminate or attenuate otic symptoms triggered or exacerbated by TMD.

Author	N° patients	Otic symptoms	% relief
Gelb et al.,1967	26	O,T,V,HL	96
Bernstein et al., 1969	28	O,T,V,HL,OF	75
Gelb et al., 1975	38	T,V	82
Rubinstein et al., 1987	68	T	41
Bush 1987	14	T	40
Kerstein 1995	23	T	83
Wright 2000	15	O,T,V	80
Kuttila et al., 2002	18	O	83
Ramirez et al., 2006	23	O,T,V,HL,OF	90

Table 3. Percentage of otic symptoms relieved by muscular relaxation oral device. O: otalgia, T: tinnitus, V: vertigo, HL: hearing-loss, OF: otic fullness.

Oral devices attempt peripheral relaxation of muscle hyperactivity triggered during anxiety and depression. These devices have been used individually or as part of varied treatment including physiotherapy, counselling, and acupuncture. However, several discrepancies limit research into this management device's methodology, making them prone to error and bias due to lack of method standardisation. This variety among methods includes the sample-size, diagnostic criteria, oral appliance, combination of oral appliance with another mode of treatment, non-validated questionnaires, absence of control group, non age and gender matching, and mailing the clinical evaluation, which makes the results difficult to interpret. The placebo effect must be considered in TMD-otic symptom treatment results. Table 3 shows otic symptom relief by single oral device treatment in TMD.[20,22,24,35,56,178,179,180] Treatment including oral devices as part of collective management were excluded due to treatment outcome non-specificity.[45,86,170,178,181,182,183,184,185,186]

10. Conclusions

Cause and effect relations between TMD and orofacial-otic symptoms are still a polemic topic. When the link is emphasized by therapeutic results the cause-effect relations get strength. Teamwork and an exhaustive symptoms assessment based on a complete structured interview and physical examination are necessary for the diagnosis and treatment of these symptoms, closing a wide conception breach existing between health disciplines.

Interdisciplinary management, including a dental specialist in craniofacial pain, offers a key tool to medical staff during these symptoms' conservative phase. Clinical success depends on each specialist's ability to study the different aspects of the same problem. One health discipline cannot always solve patients' symptomatology by themselves unless aided by the invaluable support of a multidisciplinary management team. Every specialist contributes his/her specific knowledge towards differential diagnosis addressing a correct treatment plan.

11. References

[1] Ramirez LM, Ballesteros LE, Sandoval GP. Topical Review: Temporomandibular disorders and the multmodal nature of referred otic symptoms. International Journal of Audiology 2008;47:215-27

[2] Costen, J.B. 1934. A syndrome of ear and sinus symptoms dependent upon disturbed function of the temporomandibular joint. Ann Otol;43:1-15.

[3] Myrhaug, H. 1964. The incidence of ear symptoms in cases of malocclusion and temporo-mandibular joint disturbances. Br J Oral Surg;2:28-32.

[4] Ramirez LM, Ballesteros LE, Sandoval GP. Morphological expression of disco-malleolar and anterior malleolar ligaments. A direct anatomical study. Int J Morphol 2009;27:367-79.

[5] Ramirez LM, Ballesteros LE, Sandoval GP. Tensor veli palatini and tensor tympani: Anatomical, functional and symptomatically link. Act Esp Otorrinolaringol 2010;61:26-33.

[6] Ramirez LM, Ballesteros LE, Sandoval GP. Tensor tympani muscle: Extrange chewing muscle. Med Oral Patol Oral Cir Bucal 2007;12:E96-E100

[7] Ramirez LM, Sandoval GP, Ballesteros LE, Gonzales A, Muños G. Treatment and follow up of referred otic symptomatology in 23 patients with diagnosed temporomandibular disorders. Aud Med 2006;4:73-81
[8] Lund JP, Lavigne GJ, Dubner R, Sessle BJ. Orofacial pain: From basic science to clinical management. 1st ed. Quintessence Publishing Co, Inc. Chicago, 2001
[9] Skeppar J, DDS. Treatment of craniomandibular disorders in children and young adults. J Orofacial Pain 1993;7:362-369.
[10] Youniss S, DDS. The relationship between craniomandibular disorders and otitis media in children. The J Craniomandib Pract. April 1991, Vol.9 No.2: 169-173
[11] Dao TT. Gender differences in pain. J Orofac Pain 2000;14:169-184
[12] Pergamalian A., Thomas R., Hussein Z., Greco C. The association between wear facets, bruxism, and severity of facial pain in patients with temporomandibular disorders. Journal of Prosthetic Dentistry August 2003, Vol. 90, No. 2:194-200
[13] Okeson JP ed. Management of temporomandibular disorders and occlusion. Ed 4, St. Louis: Mosby;1998. p. 149-77
[14] Major M. A controlled daytime challenge of motor performance and vigilance in sleep bruxers. J Dent Res 1999;78:1754-62
[15] Kato T, Rompre R. Sleep bruxism: and oromotor activity secondary to micro-arousal. J Dent Res 2001;80:1940-44
[16] Ware JC. Destructive bruxism: Sleep stage relationship. Sleep 1988;11:172-81
[17] Bailey DR. Tension headache and bruxism in the sleep disordered patient. Cranio 1990;8:174-82
[18] Bernhardt O, Gesch D, Schwahn C, Bitter K, Mundt T, Mack F , Kocher T, Meyer G, Hensel E, John U. Signs of temporomandibular disorders in tinnitus patients and in a population-based group of volunteers: results of the Study of Health in Pomerania. J Oral Rehabil 2004;31:311–9
[19] dos Reis AC, Hotta TH, Ferreira-Jeronymo RR, de Felicio CM, Ribeiro RF. Ear symptomatology and occlusal factors: A clinical report. J Prosthet Dent 2000;83: 21-4
[20] Bernstein JM, Mohl ND, Spiller H. Temporomandibular joint dysfunction masquerading as disease of ear, nose, and throat. Trans Am Acad Ophthalmol Otolaryngol 1969;73 1208-17
[21] Cooper BC, Cooper DL. Recognizing otolaryngologic symptoms in patients with temporomandiblar disorders. Cranio 1993;11:260-7
[22] Cooper BC, Alleva M, Cooper DL, Lucente FE. Myofacial pain dysfunction: analysis of 476 patients. Laryngoscope 1986;96:1099-2106
[23] Gelb H, Calderone JP, Gross SM, Kantor ME. The role of the dentist and the otolaryngologist in evaluating temporomandibular joint syndromes. J Prosthet Dent 1967;18: 497-503
[24] Gelb H, Arnold GE. Syndromes of the head and neck of dental origin. I. Pain caused by mandibular dysfunction. AMA Arch Otolaryngol 1959;70:681-91
[25] Keersmaekers K, De Boever JA, Van Den BL. Otalgia in patients with temporomandibular joint disorders. J Prosthet Dent 1996;75:72-6
[26] Youniss S. The relationship between craniomandibular disorders and otitis media in children. Cranio 1991;9:169-73

[27] Costen JB. A syndrome of ear and sinus symptoms dependent upon disturbed function of the temporomandibular joint. Ann Otol 1934;43:1-15
[28] Costen JB. A syndrome of ear and sinus symptoms dependent upon disturbed function of the temporomandibular joint. Ann Otol Rhinol Laryngol 1997;106:805-19
[29] Camparis CM, Formigoni G, Teixeira MJ, de Siqueira JT. Clinical evaluation of tinnitus in patients with sleep bruxism: prevalence and characteristics. J Oral Rehabil 2005;32;808-14
[30] Goodfriend DJ. Symptomatology and treatment of abnormalities of the mandibular articulation. Dent Cosmos 1933;75:844-52
[31] Ramirez LM, Ballesteros LE, Sandoval GP. Topical review: temporomandibular disorders in an integral otic symptom model. Int J Audiol 2008;47:215-27
[32] Abou-Atme YS, Zawawi KH, Melis M. Prevalence, intensity, and correlation of different TMJ symptoms in Lebanese and Italian subpopulations. J Contemp Dent Pract 2006;7:71-8
[33] Brookes GB, Maw AR, Coleman MJ. Costen's syndrome'--correlation or coincidence: a review of 45 patients with temporomandibular joint dysfunction, otalgia and other aural symptoms. Clin Otolaryngol Allied Sc 1980;5:23-36
[34] Karjalainen M, Le Bell BY, Jamsa T, Karjalainen S. Prevention of temporomandibular disorder-related signs and symptoms in orthodontically treated adolescents. A 3-year follow-up of a prospective randomized trial. Acta Odontol Scand 1997;55:319-24
[35] Bush FM. Tinnitus and otalgia in temporomandibular disorders. J Prosthet Dent 1987;58:495-8
[36] Bush FM. Tinnitus and earache: Long term studies in 105 patients with temporomandibular disorders. J Dent Res 1986;(special issue):185.
[37] Carlsson GE, Kopp S, Wedel A. Analysis of background variables in 350 patients with TMJ disorders as reported in self administered questionnaire. Community Dent Oral Epidemiol 1982;10:47-51
[38] Chole RA, Parker WS. Tinnitus and vertigo in patients with temporomandibular disorder. ArchOtolaryngol Head Neck Surg 1992;118:817-21
[39] Ciancaglini R, Loreti P, Radaelli G. Ear, nose, and throat symptoms in patients with TMD: the association of symptoms according to severity of arthropathy. J Orofac Pain 1994;8:293-97
[40] Fricton JR, Kroening R, Haley D, Siegert R. Myofascial pain syndrome of the head and neck: a review of clinical characteristics of 164 patients. Oral Surg Oral Med Oral Pathol 1985;60:615-23
[41] Gelb H, Bernstein I. Clinical evaluation of two hundred patients with temporomandibular joint syndrome". J Prosthet Dent 1983;49:234-43
[42] Gelb H, Bernstein IM. Comparison of three different populations with temporomandibular joint pain-dysfunction syndrome. Dent Clin North Am 1983;27:495-503
[43] Gelb H, Tarte J. A two-year clinical dental evaluation of 200 cases of chronic headache: the craniocervical-mandibular syndrome. J Am Dent Assoc 1975;91:1230-6
[44] Kaygusuz I, Karlidag T, Keles E, Yalcin S, Yildiz M, Alpay HC. Ear symptoms accompanying temporomandibular joint diseases. Kulak Burun Bogaz Ihtis Derg 2006;16:205-8

[45] Koskinen J, Paavolainen M, Raivio M, Roschier J. Otological manifestations in temporomandibular joint dysfunction. J Oral Rehabil 1980;7:49-54
[46] Kuttila S, Kuttila M, Le Bell BY, Alanen P, Jouko S. Aural symptoms and signs of temporomandibular disorder in association with treatment need and visits to a physician. Laryngoscope 1999;109:1669-73
[47] Luz JG, Maragno IC, Martin MC. Characteristics of chief complaints of patients with temporomandibular disorders in a Brazilian population. J Oral Rehabil 1997;4:240-3
[48] Manni A, Brunori P, Giuliani M, Modoni M, Bizzi G. Oto-vestibular symptoms in patients with temporomandibular joint dysfunction. Electromyographic study. Minerva Stomatol 1996;45:1-7
[49] Parker WS, Chole RA. Tinnitus, vertigo, and temporomandibular disorders. Am J Orthod Dentofacial Orthop 1995;107:153-8
[50] Principato JJ, Barwell DR. Biofeedback training and relaxation exercises for treatment of temporomandibular joint dysfunction. Otolaryngology 1978;86:766-9
[51] Kelly HT, Goodfriend DJ. Medical significance of equilibration of the masticating mechanism. J Prosth Dent 1960;10:496-515.
[52] Kelly HT, Goodfriend DJ. Vertigo attributable to dental and temporomandibular joint causes. J Prosthet Dent 1964;1:159-73.
[53] Wedel A, Carlsson GE. A four-year follow-up, by means of a questionnaire, of patients with functional disturbances of the masticatory system. J Oral Rehabil 1986;13:105-13
[54] Tuz HH, Onder EM, Kisnisci RS. Prevalence of otologic complaints in patients with temporomandibular disorder. Am J Orthod Dentofacial Orthop 2003;123:620-3
[55] Watanabe EK, Yatani H, Kuboki T, Matsuka Y, Terada S, Orsini MG, Yamashita A. The relationship between signs and symptoms of temporomandibular disorders and bilateral occlusal contact patterns during lateral excursions. J Oral Rehabil 1998;25:409-15
[56] Wright EF, Syms CA, Bifano SL. Tinnitus, dizziness, and nonotologic otalgia improvement through temporomandibular disorder therapy. Mil Med 2000;165:733-6
[57] D'Antonio W, Ikino C, Castro S, Balbani A, Jurado J, Bento R. Distúrbio temporo-mandibular como causa de otalgia: um estudo clínico. Rev Bras Otorrinol 2000;66:46-50.
[58] de Felicio CM, Oliveira JA, Nunes LJ, Jeronymo LF, Ferreira-Jeronymo RR. Alterações auditivas relacionadas ao zumbido nos distúrbios otológicos e da articulação temporomandibular. Rev Bras Otorrinolaringo 1999;65:141-46.
[59] de Felicio CM, Faria TG , Rodrigues da Silva MA , de Aquino AM, Junqueira CA. Temporomandibular Disorder: relationship between otologic and orofacial symptoms. Rev Bras Otorrinolaringol 2004;70:787-95.
[60] de Felício CM, Melchior Mde O, Ferreira CL, Da Silva MA. Otologic symptoms of temporomandibular disorder and effect of orofacial myofunctional therapy. Cranio 2008;26:118-25
[61] de Felício CM, de Oliveira MM, da Silva MA. Effects of orofacial myofunctional therapy on temporomandibular disorders. Cranio 2010;28:249-59
[62] Riga M, Xenellis J, Peraki E, Ferekidou E, Korres S. Aural symptoms in patients with temporomandibular joint disorders: multiple frequency tympanometry provides

objective evidence of changes in middle ear impedance. Otol Neurotol 2010;31:1359-64

[63] Pekkan G, Aksoy S, Hekimoglu C, Oghan F. Comparative audiometric evaluation of temporomandibular disorder patients with otological symptoms. J Craniomaxillofac Surg 2010;38:231-4

[64] Bernhardt O, Mundt T, Welk A, Köppl N, Kocher T, Meyer G, Schwahn C. Signs and symptoms of temporomandibular disorders and the incidence of tinnitus. J Oral Rehabil 2011; Article published online: DOI: 10.1111/j.1365-2842.2011.02224.x

[65] Bruto LH, Kós AO, Amado SM, Monteiro C, Lima MA de. Alterações otológicas nas desordens têmporo-mandibulares. Rev Bras Otorrinolaringol 2000;66:327-32.

[66] Pascoal MI, Rapoport A, Chagas JF, Pascoal MB, Costa CC, Magna LA. Prevalência dos sintomas otológicos na desordem temporomandibular: estudo de 126 casos. Rev Bras Otorrinolaringol 2001;67:627-33.

[67] Salvetti G, Manfredini D, Barsotti S, Bosco M. Otologic symptoms in temporomandibular disorders patients: is there evidence of an association-relationship?. Minerva Stomatol 2006;55:627-37

[68] Rubinstein B. Tinnitus and craniomandibular disorders--is there a link?. Swed Dent J Suppl 1993;95:1-46

[69] Lam DK, Lawrence HP, Tenenbaum HC. Aural symptoms in temporomandibular disorder patients attending a craniofacial pain unit. J Orofac Pain 2001;15:146-57

[70] Bjorne A, Agerberg G. Craniomandibular disorders in patients with Meniere's disease: a controlled study. J Orofac Pain 1996;10:28-37

[71] Lockwood AH, Salvi RJ, Coad ML, Towsley ML, Wack DS, Murphy BW. The functional neuroanatomy of tinnitus: evidence for limbic system links and neural plasticity. Neurology 1998;50:114-20

[72] Vernon J, Griest S, Press L. Attributes of tinnitus that may predict temporomandibular joint dysfunction. Cranio 1992;10:282-7

[73] Levine RA. Somatic (craniocervical) tinnitus and the dorsal cochlear nucleus hypothesis. Am J Otolaryngol 1999;20:351-62

[74] Hazell JW. Patterns of tinnitus: medical audiologic findings. J Laryngol Otol Suppl 1982;4:39-47

[75] Kuttila S, Kuttila M, Le Bell BY, Alanen P, Suonpaa J. Recurrent tinnitus and associated ear symptoms in adults. Int J Audiol 2005;44:164-70

[76] Vass Z, Shore SE, Nuttall AL, Miller JM. Direct evidence of trigeminal innervation of the cochlear blood vessels. Neuroscience 1998;84:559-67

[77] Shore SE, Vass Z, Wys NL, Altschuler RA. Trigeminal ganglion innervates the auditory brainstem. J Comp Neurol 2000;419:271-85

[78] Levine RA, Abel M, Cheng H. CNS somatosensory-auditory interactions elicit or modulate tinnitus. Exp Brain Res 2003;153:643-48

[79] Abel MD, Levine RA. Muscle contractions and auditory perception in tinnitus patients and nonclinical subjects. Cranio 2004;22:181-91

[80] Shore SE, Zhou J. Somatosensory influence on the cochlear nucleus and beyond. Hear Res 2006;216-17:90-9

[81] Young ED, Nelken I, Conley RA. Somatosensory effects on neurons in dorsal cochlear nucleus. J Neurophysiol 1995;73:743-65

[82] Kanold PO, Young ED. Proprioceptive information from the pinna provides somatosensory input to cat dorsal cochlear nucleus. J Neurosci 2001;21:7848-58
[83] Moller AR, Moller MB, Yokota M. Some forms of tinnitus may involve the extralemniscal auditory pathway. Laryngoscope 1992;102:1165-71
[84] El-Kashlan HK, Shore SE. Effects of trigeminal ganglion stimulation on the central auditory system. Hear Res 2004;189:25-30
[85] Peroz I. Otalgia and tinnitus in patients with craniomandibular dysfunctions. HNO 2001;49:713-8
[86] Sobhy OA, Koutb AR, Abdel-Baki FA, Ali TM, El Raffa RI, Khater AH. Evaluation of aural manifestations in temporo-mandibular joint dysfunction. Clin Otolaryngol Allied Sci 2004;29:382-5
[87] Kaltenbach JA, Zhang J, Finlayson P. Tinnitus as a plastic phenomenon and its possible neural underpinnings in the dorsal cochlear nucleus. Hear Res 2005;206:200-26
[88] Zhou J, Shore S. Projections from the trigeminal nuclear complex to the cochlear nuclei: a retrograde and anterograde tracing study in the guinea pig. J Neurosci Res 2004;8:901-7
[89] Kaltenbach JA. The dorsal cochlear nucleus as a participant in the auditory, attentional and emotional components of tinnitus. Hear Res 2006;216-17:224-34
[90] Lockwood AH, Salvi RJ, Burkard RF. Tinnitus. N Engl J Med 2002;347:904-10
[91] Jeanmonod D, Magnin M, Morel A. Low-threshold calcium spike bursts in the human thalamus. Common physiopathology for sensory, motor and limbic positive symptoms. Brain 1996;119:363-75
[92] Cacace AT. Expanding the biological basis of tinnitus: crossmodal origins and the role of neuroplasticity. Hear Res 2003;75:112-32
[93] Muhlnickel W, Elbert T, Taub E, Flor H. Reorganization of auditory cortex in tinnitus. Proc Natl Acad Sci USA 1998;95:10340-3
[94] Kato T, Thie NM, Huynh N, Miyawaki S, Lavigne GJ. Topical review: sleep bruxism and the role of peripheral sensory influences. J Orofac Pain 2003;17:191-213
[95] Carra MC, Rompré PH, Kato T, Parrino L, Terzano MG, Lavigne GJ, Macaluso GM. Sleep bruxism and sleep arousal: an experimental challenge to assess the role of cyclic alternating pattern. J Oral Rehabil 2011 Feb 7 [Epub ahead of print]
[96] Jastreboff PJ. Phantom auditory perception (tinnitus): mechanisms of generation and perception. Neurosci Res 1990;8:221-54
[97] Proctor B. Embryology and anatomy of the eustachian tube. Arch Otolaryngol 1967;86:503-14
[98] Strickland EM, Hanson JR, Anson BJ. Branchial sources of auditory oscicles in man. I. Literature. Arch Otolaryngol 1962;76:100-22
[99] Rodriguez Vazquez JF, Merida V, Jimenez CJ. A study of the os goniale in man. Acta Anat (Basel) 1991;142:188-92
[100] Rodriguez Vazquez JF, Merida V, Jimenez CJ. Relationships between the temporomandibular joint and the middle ear in human fetuses. J Dent Res 1993;72:62-6
[101] Yuodelis RA. The morphogenesis of the human temporomandibular joint and its associated structures. J Dent Res 1966;45:182-91

[102] Thilander B, Carlsson GE, Ingervall B. Postnatal development of the human temporomandibular joint. I. A histological study. Acta Odontol Scand 1976;34:117-26

[103] Arlen H. The otomandibular syndrome: a new concept. Ear Nose Throat J 1977;56:60-2

[104] Salen B, Zakrisson JE. Electromyogram of the tensor tympani muscle in man during swallowing. Acta Otolaryngol 1978;85:453-5

[105] Ramirez LM, Ballesteros LE, Sandoval GP. Tensor veli palatini and tensor tympani muscles: anatomical, functional, and symptomatic links. Acta Otorrinolaringol Esp 2010;61:26-33

[106] Zipfel TE, Kaza SR, Greene JS. Middle-ear myoclonus. J Laryngol Otol 2000;114:207-9

[107] Pau HW, Punke C, Zehlicke T, Dressler D, Sievert U. Tonic contractions of the tensor tympani muscle: a key to some non-specific middle ear symptoms? Hypothesis and data from temporal bone experiments. Acta Otolaryngol 2005;125:1168-75

[108] Chan SW, Reade PC. Tinnitus and temporomandibular pain-dysfunction disorder", Clin Otolaryngol Allied Sci 1994;19:370-80

[109] Kamerer DB. Electromyographic correlation of tensor tympani and tensor veli palatini muscles in man. Laryngoscope 1978;88:651-62

[110] Jung HH, Han SH, Nam SY, Kim YH, Kim JI. Myosin heavy chain composition of rat middle ear muscles. Acta Otolaryngol 2004;24:569-73

[111] Van den Berge H, kingma H, kluge C, Marres EH. Electrophysiological aspects of the middle ear muscle reflex in the rat: latency, rise time and effect on sound transmission. Hear Res 1990;48:209-19

[112] Ochi K, Ohashi T, Kinoshita H. Acoustic tensor tympani response and vestibular-evoked myogenic potential. Laryngoscope 2002;112:2225-9

[113] Malkin DP. The role of TMD dysfunction in the etiology of middle ear diseases. Int J Orthod 1987;25:21-1

[114] Klockhoff I, Anderson H. Reflex activity in the tensor tympani muscle recorded in man; preliminary report. Acta Otolaryngol 1960;51:184-8

[115] Ogutcen-Toller MO, Juniper RP. Audiological evaluation of the aural symptoms in temporomandibular joint dysfunction. J Craniomaxillofac Surg 1993;21:2-8

[116] Dolowitz DA, Ward JW, Fingerle CO, Smith CC. The role of muscular incoordination in the pathogenesis of the temporomandibular joint syndrome. Laryngoscope 1964;74:790-801

[117] Goto TK, Yahagi M, Nakamura Y, Tokumori K, Langenbach GE, Yoshiura K. In vivo cross-sectional area of human jaw muscles varies with section location and jaw position. J Dent Res 2005;84:570-5

[118] Sehhati-Chafai-Leuwer S, Wenzel S, Bschorer R, Seedorf H, Kucinski T, Maier H, Leuwer R. Pathophysiology of the Eustachian tube--relevant new aspects for the head and neck surgeon. J Craniomaxillofac Surg 2006;34:351-4

[119] Sharav Y, Tzukert A, Refaeli B. Muscle pain index in relation to pain, dysfunction, and dizziness associated with the myofascial pain-dysfunction syndrome. Oral Surg Oral Med Oral Pathol 1978;46:742-7

[120] Henderson DH, Cooper JC, Bryan GW, Van Sickels JE. Otologic complaints in temporomandibular joint syndrome. Arch Otolaryngol Head Neck Surg 1992;118:1208-13

[121] Penkner K, Kole W, Kainz J, Schied G, Lorenzoni M. The function of tensor veli palatini muscles in patients with aural symptoms and temporomandibular disorder. An EMG study. J Oral Rehabil 2000;27:344-8
[122] McDonnell JP, Needleman HL, Charchut S, Allred EN, Roberson DW, Kenna MA, Jones D. The relationship between dental overbite and eustachian tube dysfunction. Laryngoscope 2001;111:310-16
[123] Azadani PN, Jafarimehr E, Shokatbakhsh A, Pourhoseingholi MA, Ghougeghi A. The effect of dental overbite on eustachian tube dysfunction in Iranian children. Int J Pediatr Otorhinolaryngol 2007;71:325-31
[124] Holborow C. Eustachian tubal function: changes throughout childhood and neuro-muscular control. J Laryngol Otol 1975;89:47-55
[125] Marasa FK, Ham BD. Case reports involving the treatment of children with chronic otitis media with effusion via craniomandibular methods. Cranio 1988;6:256-70
[126] Barsoumian R, Kuehn DP, Moon JB, Canady JW. An anatomic study of the tensor veli palatini and dilatator tubae muscles in relation to eustachian tube and velar function. Cleft Palate Craniofac J 1988;35:101-10
[127] Rood SR, Doyle WJ. Morphology of tensor veli palatini, tensor tympani, and dilatator tubae muscles. Ann Otol Rhinol Laryngol 1978;87:202-10
[128] Rood SR. The morphology of M. tensor veli palatini in the five-month human fetus. Am J Anat 1973;138:191-5
[129] Kierner AC, Mayer R, Kirschhofer K. Do the tensor tympani and tensor veli palatini muscles of man form a functional unit? A histochemical investigation of their putative connections. Hear Res 2002;165:48-52
[130] Eriksson PO, Zafar H, Haggman-Henrikson B. Deranged jaw-neck motor control in whiplash-associated disorders. Eur J Oral Sci 2004;112:25-32
[131] de Wijer WA, Steenks MH, de Leeuw L, Bosman F, Helders PJ. Symptoms of the cervical spine in temporomandibular and cervical spine disorders. J Oral Rehabil 1996;23:742-50
[132] Loughner BA, Larkin LH, Mahan PE. Nerve entrapment in the lateral pterygoid muscle. Oral Surg Oral Med Oral Pathol 1990;69:299-306
[133] Williamson EH. Interrelationship of internal derangements of the temporomandibular joint, headache, vertigo, and tinnitus: a survey of 25 patients. Cranio 1990;8:301-6
[134] Pinto OF. A new structure related to the temporomandibular joint and middle ear. J Prosthet Dent 1962;12:95-103
[135] Komori E, Sugisaki M, Tanabe H, Katoh S. Discomalleolar ligament in the adult human. Cranio 1986;4:299-305
[136] Loughner BA, Larkin LH, Mahan PE. Discomalleolar and anterior malleolar ligaments: possible causes of middle ear damage during temporomandibular joint surgery. Oral Surg Oral Med Oral Pathol 1989;68:14-22
[137] Ioannides CA, Hoogland GA. The disco-malleolar ligament: a possible cause of subjective hearing loss in patients with temporomandibular joint dysfunction. J Maxillofac Surg 1983;11:227-31
[138] Coleman RD. Temporomandibular joint: relation of the retrodiskal zone to Meckel's cartilage and lateral pterygoid muscle. J Dent Res 1970;49:626-30
[139] Morgan DH, Goode RL, Christiansen RL, Tiner LW. The TMJ-ear connection. Cranio 1995;13:42-3

[140] Ogutcen-Toller MO, Keskin M. Computerized 3-dimensional study of the embryologic development of the human masticatory muscles and temporomandibular joint. J Oral Maxillofac Surg 2000;58;1381-6

[141] Merida V, Rodriguez Vazquez JF, Jimenez CJ. Anterior tympanic artery: course, ramification and relationship with the temporomandibular joint. Acta Anat (Basel) 1997;158:222-26

[142] Perry HT, Xu Y, Forbes DP. The embryology of the temporomandibular joint. Cranio 1985;3:125-32

[143] Rodriguez-Vazquez JF, Merida-Velasco JR, Merida-Velasco JA, Jimenez-Collado J. Anatomical considerations on the discomalleolar ligament. J Anat 1998;192:617-21

[144] Sencimen M, Yalçin B, Doğan N, Varol A, Okçu KM, Ozan H, Aydintuğ YS. Anatomical and functional aspects of ligaments between the malleus and the temporomandibular joint. Int J Oral Maxillofac Surg 2008;37:943-7

[145] Burch JG. The cranial attachment of the sphenomandibular (tympanomandibular) ligament. Anat Rec 1966;156:433-7

[146] Alkofide EA, Clark E, el-Bermani W, Kronman JH, Mehta N. The incidence and nature of fibrous continuity between the sphenomandibular ligament and the anterior malleolar ligament of the middle ear. J Orofac Pain 1997;11:7-14

[147] Ogutcen-Toller M. The morphogenesis of the human discomalleolar and sphenomandibular ligaments. J Craniomaxillofac Surg 1995;23:42-6

[148] Rodriguez Vazquez JF, Merida Velasco JR, Jimenez Collado J. Development of the human sphenomandibular ligament. Anat Rec 1992;233:453-60

[149] Ramirez LM, Ballesteros LE, Sandoval GP. Morphological expression of disco-malleolar and anterior malleolar ligaments. A direct anatomical study. Int J Morphol 2009;27:367-79

[150] Eckerdal O. The petrotympanic fissure: a link connecting the tympanic cavity and the temporomandibular joint. Cranio 1991;9:15-22

[151] Kim HJ, Jung HS, Kwak HH, Shim KS, Hu KS, Park HD, Park HW, Chung IH. The discomallear ligament and the anterior ligament of malleus: an anatomic study in human adults and fetuses. Surg Radiol Anat 2004;26:39-45

[152] Cheynet F, Guyot L, Richard O, Layoun W, Gola R. Discomallear and malleomandibular ligaments: anatomical study and clinical applications. Surg Radiol Anat 2003;25:152-7

[153] Rodriguez Vazquez JF, Merida V, Jimenez CJ. Development of the human sphenomandibular ligament. Anat Rec 1992;233:453-60

[154] Libin B. The cranial mechanism and its dental implications. Int J Orthod 1984;22:7-11

[155] Johansson, A.S., Isberg, A. & Isacsson, G. (1990).A radiographic and histologic study of the topographic relations in the temporomandibular joint region: implications for a nerve entrapment mechanism. J Oral Maxillofac Surg, 48, 953-961.

[156] Myers, L.J. (1988). Possible inflammatory pathways relating temporomandibular joint dysfunction to otic symptoms. Cranio, 6, 64-70.

[157] Tonndorf J, Khanna SM. Tympanic-membrane vibrations in human cadaver ears studied by time-averaged holography. J Acoust Soc Am 1972;52:1221-33

[158] Sun Q, Gan RZ, Chang KH, Dormer KJ. Computer integrated finite element modeling of human middle ear. Biomech Model Mechanobiol 2002;1:109-22

[159] Dalhoff E, Turcanu D, Zenner HP, Gummer AW. Distortion product otoacoustic emissions measured as vibration on the eardrum of human subjects. PNAS 2007;104:1546-51
[160] Bekesy GV. Experiments in Hearing. New York, McGraw-Hill, 1960
[161] Koike T, Wada H, Kobayashi T. Modeling of the human middle ear using the finite-element method. J. Acoust Soc Am 2002;111:1306-17
[162] Wada H, Ando M, Takeuchi M, Sugawara H, Koike T, Kobayashi T, Hozawa K, Gemma T, Nara M. Vibration measurement of the tympanic membrane of guinea pig temporal bones using time-averaged speckle pattern interferometry. J Acoust Soc Am 2002;111:2189-99
[163] Sato I, Arai H, Asaumi R, Imura K, Kawai T, Yosue T. Classifications of tunnel-like structure of human petrotympanic fissure by cone beam CT. Surg Radiol Anat 2008:30:323-6
[164] Nakajima HH, Ravicz ME, Rosowski JJ, Peake WT, Merchant SN. Experimental and clinical studies of malleus fixation. Laryngoscope 2005;115:147-54
[165] Zhao F, Wada H, Koike T, Ohyama K, Kawase T, Stephens D. Middle ear dynamic characteristics in patients with otosclerosis. Ear Hear 2002;23:150-8
[166] Huber A, Koike T, Wada H, Nandapalan V, Fisch U. Fixation of the anterior mallear ligament: diagnosis and consequences for hearing results in stapes surgery. Ann Otol Rhinol Laryngol 2003;112:348-55
[167] Cheng T, Gan RZ. Mechanical properties of anterior malleolar ligament from experimental measurement and material modeling analysis. Biomech Model Mechanobiol 2008;7:387-94
[168] Morgan DH. Tinnitus of TMJ origin: a preliminary report. Cranio 1992;10:124-29
[169] Ren YF, Isberg A. Tinnitus in patients with temporomandibular joint internal derangement. Cranio 1995;13:75-80
[170] Wright EF, Bifano SL. Tinnitus improvement through TMD therapy. J Am Dent Assoc 1997;128:1424-32
[171] Abe S, Ouchi Y, Ide Y, Yonezu H. Perspectives on the role of the lateral pterygoid muscle and the sphenomandibular ligament in temporomandibular joint function. Cranio 1997;15:203-7
[172] Ouchi Y, Abe S, Sun-Ki R, Agematsu H, Watanabe H et al. Attachment of the sphenomandibular ligament to bone during intrauterine embryo development for the control of mandibular movement. Bull Tokyo Dent Coll 1998;39:91-4
[173] Burch JG.Activity of the accessory ligaments of the temporomandibular joint. J Prosthet Dent 1970;24:621-8
[174] Merida-Velasco JR, Rodriguez-Vazquez JF, Merida-Velasco JA, Jimenez-Collado J. The vascular relationship between the temporomandibular joint and the middle ear in the human fetus. J Oral Maxillofac Surg 1999;57:146-53
[175] Scolozzi P, Becker M, Richter M. Temporomandibular joint osteoarthritis: a cause of a serous otitis media? A case report. J Oral Maxillofac Surg 2004;62:97-100
[176] Regev E, Koplewitz BZ, Nitzan DW, Bar-Ziv J. Ankylosis of the temporomandibular joint as a sequela of septic arthritis and neonatal sepsis. Pediatr Infect Dis J 2003;22.99-101

[177] Takes RP, Langeveld AP, Baatenburg de Jong RJ. Abscess formation in the temporomandibular joint as a complication of otitis media. J Laryngol Otol 2000;114:373-5
[178] Rubinstein B, Carlsson GE. Effects of stomatognathic treatment on tinnitus: a retrospective study. Cranio 1987;5:254-9
[179] Ramirez LM, Sandoval GP, Ballesteros LE, Gonzales A, Muños G. Treatment and follow up of referred otic symptomatology in 23 patients with diagnosed temporomandibular disorders. Aud Med 2006;4:73-81
[180] Kuttila M, Le Bell Y, Savolainen-Niemi E, Kuttila S, Alanen P. Efficiency of occlusal appliance therapy in secondary otalgia and temporomandibular disorders. Acta Odontol Scand 2002;60:248-54
[181] Bjorne, A. & Agerberg, G. (2003a). Reduction in sick leave and costs to society of patients with Meniere's disease after treatment of temporomandibular and cervical spine disorders: a controlled six-year cost-benefit study. Cranio, 21, 136-43.
[182] Bjorne, A. & Agerberg, G. (2003b). Symptom relief after treatment of temporomandibular and cervical spine disorders in patients with Meniere's disease: a three-year follow-up. Cranio, 21, 50-60
[183] Erlandsson, S.I., Rubinstein, B. & Carlsson, S.G. (1991). Tinnitus: evaluation of biofeedback and stomatognathic treatment. Br J Audiol, 25:151-61.
[184] Kerstein RB. Treatment of myofascial pain dysfunction syndrome with occlusal therapy to reduce lengthy disclusion time--a recall evaluation. Cranio 1995;13:105-15
[185] Tullberg M, Ernberg M. Long-term effect on tinnitus by treatment of temporomandibular disorders: a two-year follow-up by questionnaire. Acta Odontol Scand 2006;64:89-96
[186] Kaygusuz I, Karlidag T, Keles E, Yalcin S, Yildiz M et al. Ear symptoms accompanying temporomandibular joint diseases. Kulak Burun Bogaz Ihtis Derg 2006;16:205-8

Part 3

Somatic Tinnitus

4

Tinnitus School – An Integrated Management of Somatic Tinnitus

D. Alpini[1] A. Cesarani[2] and A. Hahn[3]
[1]*Sc. Institute S. Maria Nascente, "Don Carlo Gnocchi" Foundation, Milan,*
[2]*Audiology Institute University of Milan, Milan,*
[3]*ENT Clinic, 3rd Medical Faculty, Charles University Prague, Prague,*
[1,2]*Italy*
[3]*Czech Republic*

1. Introduction

Epidemiological data suggest that tinnitus is something more and something different from an auditory symptom. In fact, subjective tinnitus is reported to be present in 10-15% (Axelson et. al 1995) persons in general population but it represents a medical problem, that interferes with general and emotional health state, only about 2%. Furthermore, factors associated with tinnitus such as hearing loss, hypertension, hormonal disorders, anxiety, depression are more frequent than tinnitus itself. (Sindhusake et al. 2004)

Stress is known to be a significant factor influencing the clinical course of tinnitus. Auditory system is in fact particularly sensitive to the effects of different stress factors (chemical, oxidative, emotional, ...). Horner in 2003 described different stages of auditory pathways reacting to stress: alarm, resistance and exhaustion. Individual characteristics of stress reaction may explain different aspects of tinnitus in various patients with different responses to treatment, despite similar audiological and aetiological factors. A model based on individual reactions to stress factors (Stress Reaction Tinnitus - SRT -Model) could explain tinnitus as an alarm signal. In 2007 Alpini et al. described a therapeutic proposal based on SRT Model, through an integrated approach to the management of patients suffering from chronic tinnitus. The educational aspect was emphasized and therefore the approach was named Tinnitus School, that is a three-phases program (counselling, training, home training) mainly based on fitted physiotherapeutic protocol.

The usefulness of physical exercises in Tinnitus patients for reducing the emotional arousal that is underlined by different Authors, e.g ranging from Dehler et al. (2000) to Biesenger et al. (2010), but, in our experience, fitted physical activity could be the specific treatment of Somatic Tinnitus.

Somatic tinnitus regards a sub-group of tinnitus suffers. It is defined as tinnitus which is associated to a somatic disorder involving the head and the neck. Dehmel et al. (2008) introduced the Somatic Tinnitus Syndrome (STS). They presented the anatomical basis for the auditory-somatosensory interactions and showed how auditory neurons respond to somatosensory stimulation. Particularly, muscle--skeletal system could be a chronic stress source. In this way muscle-skeletal disorders can pathologically integrate with auditory disturbances increasing tinnitus. In this way, Stress Reaction Tinnitus (SRT) model could be implemented into Somatic Tinnitus Syndrome (STS) model and Tinnitus School can act through fitted physiotherapy aimed to a patient-oriented treatment of selected tinnitus patients.

2. Tinnitus school in somatic tinnitus treatment

2.1 Stress reaction tinnitus model

In short-term stress reaction, hypothalamus plays an essential role in the integration of stress responses (alarm phase) through the connection between brainstem and spinal cord sympathetic and parasympathetic centres. In long-term stress, the same activation can be damaging via the prolonged secretion of stress hormones (exhaustion phase). Individual characteristics of stress reaction may explain different aspects of tinnitus in different patients, and different responses to treatment, despite similar audiological and aetiological factors.

For severe disabling chronic tinnitus, Shulman in 1995 and 2002 demonstrated that a final common pathway exists in the medial temporal lobe system, being its basic process the establishment of a paradoxical auditory memory. He proposed a model for tinnitus in which the final common pathway involves hippocampus and cerebellum providing the neurochemical basis (hippocampus) and the cognitive and motor basis (cerebellum) of behavioural aspects of tinnitus. Furthermore, Zenner & Zalaman in 2004 showed that in chronic tinnitus patients attention is pathologically shifted toward tinnitus and, in this way, cognitive functions are disturbed. The importance of limbic-auditory interaction in Tinnitus generation have been highlighted by Rauschercker at al (2010). According to the Authors limbic and auditory brain areas interact at the thalamic level and tinnitus can be tuned out by feedback connections from limbic regions which block the tinnitus signal from reaching auditory cortex. If the limbic region is dysfunctional because of chronic overloading stress (emotional tagging), this "noise- cancellation" mechanism breaks down and chronic severe disabling tinnitus results

In SRT model tinnitus may become an alarm signal, just like an "alarm bell", at least at its onset (Alpini & Cesarani, 2006); tinnitus could become a disabling symptom only in subjects chronically exposed to stress factors which are unable to switch off the alarm signal and to counteract the effect of the stressors. Individual ability to counteract stress factors is in fact strictly specific for each subject: this means that the evolution from alarm to exhaustion is specific for each patient. Therefore, the definition of "acute" or "chronic" tinnitus cannot be referred to a standardized time period but has to be fitted to each subject: generally speaking, acute tinnitus may be correlated to the stress alarm phase, chronic tinnitus to the resistance stress phase, and chronic severe disabling tinnitus may correspond to the exhaustion phase. According to this model, stress signals of a specific patient have to be identified during the "alarm" phase in order to prevent an evolution toward a resistance phase and, especially, an exhaustion phase. These phases lead to chronic disabling tinnitus in which the emotional-affective activation is dominant.

In 2011 Bergado et al. proposed the 'emotional tag' concept, according to which the activation of the amygdala by emotionality would result in the modulation of neural plasticity in brain regions (e.g. hippocampus) involved in shaping memory of the emotional event. The 'synaptic tag' model explain the specificity of synaptic plasticity and it could represent the effects of the 'emotional tag' on synaptic plasticity in the hippocampus. In Somatic Tinnitus factors such as intensity, duration of sensory-motor distress and controllability of the emotional experience, age of exposure should be taken into account.

These factors do not only affect the behavioural outcome of the stressful experience but also find their expression in varieties in the neuronal and biochemical pathways that are activated, and in the way those will interact with memory formation mechanisms leading to the "paradoxical auditory memory"(Cluny et al 2004). In this way, the removal of stress factors is necessary for general health condition and is the prerequisite to cognitive-behaviour treatments (CBT). CBT is proposed in order to promote behavioural re-organization helping the patient to cope with tinnitus, according to the view that tinnitus is a systemic problem stemming from imbalance in the excitatory and inhibitory inputs to auditory neurons (Kaltenbach, 2010, Vanneste et al. 2010).
We combine accurate anamnesis and Feldman masking test (1971) with psychometric questionnaires in order to determine the individual phase of stress reaction. In our experience the Tinnitus Reaction Questionnaire (TRQ, Wilson et al. 1991) is useful to identify the stress phase (acute, resistance, exhaustion) of a specific patient. TRQ is a self-reported scale designed to assess perceived distress associated with tinnitus. It is composed of 26 items describing some of the potential effects of tinnitus on lifestyle, general well-being, and emotional state. Respondents are asked to rate the extent to which each of the potential effects have applied to them over the last week on a 5 point scale (0: not at all; 4: almost all the time). Respondents are also asked to indicate how frequently tinnitus induces some reactions such as depression, anger, confusion (from not at all to always). The total score ranges from 0 to 104. A lower score represents slight reaction to tinnitus (alarm) while higher scores indicate deeply negative reaction (exhaustion).
Regarding stressor identification we adopted a modified CAPPE questionnaire (Nodar, 1996) combined with an accurate evaluation of patient general medical documentation. CAPPE questionnaire investigates the presence of different kind of stressors: Chemical (prolonged expositions to solvents, assumptions of ototoxic drugs), Acoustic (noise exposure, acoustic neuroma, otosclerosis, hearing loss), Pathologies (diabetes, thyroiditis, autoimmune diseases), Physical (professional stress, worsening of tinnitus during physical exercises), and Emotional (sleep disorders, job change, depression).

2.1.1 Tinnitus as a motor system alarm

Somatic Tinnitus occurs when the patient feels the effect of head and neck muscle contractions on changing the intensity of the quality of tinnitus, for instance during clenching the teeth or head rotation. In these cases, tinnitus is modulated by stimuli of the somatosensory system as a result of muscle contractions. This is not surprising because the auditory system is part of the most complex sensory-motor system involved in the head position regulation, necessary to provide gravitation reference, prerequisite for a correct orientation of the human subject in the environment. The brainstem and cerebellum are the main sites of integration of multi-sensorial information from the inner ear, retina and proprioceptors regarding head position, body position, gravity, visual landmarks and movement of the jaw, the tongue, and the pharynx. (Simmons et al 2008, Norena, 2010). In a simple experiment Jousmäki and Hari (1998) described how auditory input can modulate or even determine the touch sensation. Subjects were asked to rub their hands and the thereby evoked sounds were played back to them. When the high frequency content of the played back signals increased, the subjects felt the skin on their palms becoming dry as parchment paper. This so called parchment-skin illusion is an impressive example of auditory-somatosensory integration. The converse was shown by Levine et al. (2007): forceful manipulations or contractions of the muscles of jaw, head or neck elicited the perception in

58% of the subjects. Several studies have demonstrated the interactions between the somatosensory and auditory system at the dorsal cochlear nucleus (DCN) (Tyler et al. 2008, Vanneste et al 2010, Yang et al. 2010), inferior colliculus, and parietal association areas. In particular, auditory and somatosensory (proprioceptive and tactile) pathways converge into specialized multisensory brain areas, particularly right inferior frontal gyrus and both right and left insula, that work as multisensory operators for the processing of stimulus identity (Renier et al. 2009).

2.2 Tinnitus school

Tinnitus School is aimed to promote behavioural re-organization by helping the patient to cope with tinnitus decreasing paradoxical memory and improving diversion and distraction of auditory attention. The organization model of Tinnitus School, physical exercise integrated in an educational program, is like to that of the well-known Back School (Tavafina et al. 2007). Treatment is based on three phases: Counselling, Training, Home Training. In somatic tinnitus treatment, Tinnitus School is especially paid to sensory-motor system through three steps of treatment:

1. removing cervico-cephalic sensory-motor disturbances, by means of Manual Medicine techniques (Maigne & Nieves, 2005)
2. leading the patient to an awareness of his/her own body and learning breath and neck tension control, through physical exercises
3. shifting patient attention away from tinnitus, thorough home physical exercises

2.2.1 Counselling

Counselling is carried out by the physician who visited the patient and prepared the treatment planning. Firstly the physician explains the main aspects of the Auditory system stressing patient attention to the phenomena involved in chronic tinnitus: paradoxical auditory memory and pathological attention to tinnitus. Lifestyle and drug assumption are investigated in order to identify specific stress factors and possibilities of changing are discussed with the patient. Perceived stress was quantified through Perceived Stress Questionnaire (PSQ) (Fliege et al. 2005). It is designed to represent the subjective perspective of the individual ("You feel... "). Because stress results from overload of experienced unpredictability and uncontrollability of events, the existence of stress in a subject is partially inferred from information on the person's experience of lack of control. The presented stress experiences in PSQ were intended to be abstract enough to be applicable to adults of any age, stage of life, sex, or occupation, but at the same time interpretable as specific to a variety of real-life situations. For example, "you feel under pressure from deadlines" could refer to anything ranging from a payment, to an oncoming birthday party, or to a grant proposal. This questionnaire asks the respondent how often does certain experiences of stress occurred in the last month. The content of the items is not referred to tinnitus but it focuses on a more cognitive appraisal of stress. PSQ is a 20-item questionnaire of 4 scales with 5 items each resulted:

- Scale 1 (worries) covers worries, anxious concerns for the future, and feelings of desperation and frustration (e.g "you have many worries")
- Scale 2 (tension) explores tense disquietude, exhaustion, and the lack of relaxation (e.g. "you feel mentally exhausted")

- Scale 3 (joy) is concerned with positive feelings of challenge, joy, energy, and security (e.g." you are full of energy") .
- Scale 4 (demands) covers perceived environmental demands, such as lack of time, pressure, and overload (e.g "you feel you are in a hurry") .

  Each positive (Yes) answer to scales 1-2-4 is scored 1. Joy scale is score 1 for each negative (No) answer because all items of this scale are positively worded. Thus maximum possible score, that to say the most unbearable stress perception, is 20 : the higher the total score is, the higher the perceived stress.

During Counselling phase the physician performs an accurate evaluation of posture, temporo-mandibular joints (TMJs) (Riga M et al, 2010) and cervical spine, in order to remove the main somatosensorial trigger and tender points in the cervico-cephalic district that can be interpreted as connected to chronic tinnitus generation.

Trigger points are described as hyperirritable spots in skeletal muscle that are associated with palpable nodules in taut bands of muscle fibres. Trigger points are small contraction knots and a common cause of pain. Compression of a trigger point may elicit local tenderness, referred pain, or local twitch response. It is common to induce transient tinnitus when stimulating trigger points in trapezius muscle. More specifically, somatic tinnitus suffers frequently present modulation of their spontaneous tinnitus during appropriate stimulation of trigger points in cervical and shoulder muscles. A tender point hurts to the touch and causes some degree of pain in that area, while a trigger point may not necessarily be painful to the touch but causes a degree of pain (or tinnitus in this specific field of investigation) to be felt in another area.

Manual Medicine treatment of tinnitus suffering is thus integrated with physical exercises of the Tinnitus School program, including also High Velocity Low Amplitude vertebral manipulations, directly performed by the physician.

Counselling is completed by modified bibliotherapy. Self-help books exist for a wide variety of psychological problems. Studies of their value indicate that they can help individuals to make substantial improvements (Malouff et al. 2010), on average about as much as psychotherapy. We propose to our patient selected Italian translated lectures from "Tinnitus: A Self-Management Guide for the Ringing in Your Ears". This self-help book by Henry & Wilson (2001) is based on cognitive–behavioural principles, including educational information on tinnitus, cognitive reappraisal and restructuring, relaxation and stress management techniques, attention control techniques, use of self-instruction, making lifestyle changes, and maintaining gains.

2.2.2 Training

Training is performed by a physiotherapist, in a gymnasium, in a small class of patients (3 subjects). Class treatment improve comparison and cooperation between patients and improve positive enforcement.

Tinnitus School is constituted by ten sessions subdivided into three sessions per week along two weeks followed by two sessions per week along two other weeks.

The first step is to prepare the patient to cooperate in a complex program involving movement, thinking and learning. Muscle-skeletal impairments are often provoked or associated to tension and anxiety, that is why head and neck disorders have to be treated before training. Furthermore, it is more necessary to begin treatment with simple relaxation exercises. (Weber et al. 2002) to manage patient's tension.

Physical Exercises are pointed to postural control because, in chronic somatic Tinnitus the abnormal alignment of body parts with respect to each other and to the base of support may be due both to musculoskeletal cervico-cephalic impairments and changes in patient's internal perception of the own sensations induced by pathological attention to tinnitus.
Simple exercises have to be planned and they are generally pointed to mobilization of the pelvis, of the cervical rachis and the thoraco-lumbar spine. In some cases massages can be useful either to relax the patient or to mobilize joints, including Slow Velocity High Amplitude vertebral manipulations performed by the physiotherapist.

Tinnitus school gymnasium training protocol

Supine (all the exercise are performed having patients' head comfortably lying on a pillow)

- Relaxation exercises with control of breathing improving consciousness of abdominal or thorax breathing: deep inhaling followed, after few seconds, by a forced exhaling pronouncing the word "one". This exercises is repeated 8-10 times
- Patients move the head, first slowly and then faster, in all directions focusing a target straight on the ceiling
- Patients take the right knee against the chest, then extend the leg and take the left knee against the chest. A gentle traction of the flexed knee is performed by patient himself when the knee is taken against the chest
- Patients take both knees to the chest, contemporarily, helping, gently, with the hands
- Patients lift pelvis taking contemporarily the arms extended over the head. Then patients re-take arms along the body lowering the pelvis
- Patients grasp a stick. Then they extend the arms over the head and then return in primary position
- In the quadrupedal position, patients inhale and arch the back taking the head between the arms. Then they exhale while retro-flexing the head and rotating the pelvis in hyperlordosis
- In quadrupedal position, patients extend contemporary the right arm and the left leg. Then repeat with the left arm and the right leg
- In prone position, patients lift their left arm and the right leg maintaining the forehead over the bed. Then they repeat with the right arm and the left leg

Sitting

- Patients move the head first slowly and then faster in all directions focusing on a target straight in front
- Patients look to for three targets sited, respectively, in front, at their left and at their right. Then patients focus on the front target, then they move the head focusing on the right-sited target. At last they rotate leftward the head maintaining the focus on the right-sited target
- Patients focus on the frontal target. Then they move the head leftward and focus on the left-sited target. At last they rotate rightward the head maintaining the focus on the left-sited target
- Patients turn the head rightward and focus on a target on the lateral wall. Then they take the head straight maintaining focusing, through eyes counter-rotation, and count until 10
- Patients turn the head leftward and focus on a target on the lateral wall. Then they take the head straight maintaining focus on the target, through eyes counter-rotation, and count until 10

- Patients extend the right arm and lift their thumb. Thus patients move slowly the arm to-and-from before along an horizontal direction and then along a vertical direction. Patients pursuit the thumb with eyes only, first slowly and then increasing progressively the velocity of thumb displacement
- As above but moving contemporarily also the head trying to maintain the eyes still
- Patients grasp a stick with both hands and take the stick behind the shoulder positioning the stick at level of cervico-dorsal junction. In this position they rotate to-and-fro the trunk maintaining the head still also focusing on a target straight in front. Rotation of the trunk have to be harmonic with quiet breathing
- Patients put the stick forward on the sternum at the level of the sterno-clavear joint. Then they perform rhythmic backward displacements of shoulders
- In this position they rotate to-and-fro the trunk maintaining the head still also through fixation of a target straight in front. Rotation of the trunk have to be harmonic with quiet breathing
- Paying attention to quiet breathing patients inspire. Then, exhaling, they bend forward taking the head on the right knee. They wait 10 seconds. Then, inhaling they return in sitting position.
- Paying attention to quiet breathing patients inspire. Then, exhaling they bend forward taking the head on the left knee. They wait 10 seconds. Then, inhaling they return in sitting position.
- Patients Inhale. Exhaling they bend forward to keep an object on the floor. Then they inhale and take it up over the head and then they fixate it for 10 seconds. Patients inhale. Exhaling they bend forward and take the object on the floor

Standing

- Patients focus themselves on a mirror and align correctly their posture. Thus they maintain quiet equilibrium for 1 minute, paying attention to breathing; at first they maintain eyes open and successively they close the eyes imagining the correct position in their mind. They remain in this position for at least 1 minute paying attention to breathing. Then they oscillate to-and-fro according to the breath rhythm, hearing the air that enter and then exits from the lungs
- Patients in quiet upright position fixate a target on a mirror. In this case they have two planes of fixation: the target and their image. Thus they have to be able to extract the correct fixation information from visual inputs. Then they oscillate to-and-fro according to the breath rhythm hearing the air that enter and then exits from the lungs
- Patients keep a little object and lift it over the head fixating it. Then they deeply inspire. Expiring, they bend forward taking the object on the floor. They wait 10 seconds and then, inspiring, they lift again the object over the head
- Patients take a little object over their head. Fixating the object they move it in small circles according to breath rhythm hearing the air that enter and then exits from the lungs

2.2.3 Home training

As in every "school" , home training is as important as class training. A part of gymnasium session is dedicated to instruct patients how to correctly perform home exercises. Home protocol is showed in Tab II. Exercises have to be performed every day twice a day.

Tinnitus school home training protocol

Supine

- Relaxation exercises with control of breathing, improving consciousness of abdominal or thorax breathing: deep inhale followed, after few seconds, by a forced exhale pronouncing the word "one". This exercises is repeated 8-10 times
- Take your two knees to the chest, contemporary, helping, gently, with the hands
- Lift your pelvis taking contemporary your arms extended over your head. Then re-take your arms along the body lowering your pelvis
- Grasp a stick. Take your extended arms over your head and then return in primary position
- In prone position lift your left arm and the right leg maintaining your forehead over the bed. Then repeat with the right arm and the left leg.

Sitting

- Move your head first slowly and then faster in all directions focusing on a target straight in front of you
- Grasp a stick with both hands and take the stick behind the shoulder positioning the stick at the level of the cervico-dorsal junction. In this position rotate to-and-fro the trunk maintaining the head still also through fixation of a target straight in front. Rotation of the trunk have to be harmonic with quiet breathing
- Repeat the exercise putting the stick forward on the sternum at the level of the sterno-clavear joint. Then perform rhythmic backward displacements of shoulders

Standing

- With your hands on a table, lift yourself on your tiptoes, maintain this position for 30 seconds. Pay attention to breathing!
- With your hands on a table, lift yourself on your heels, maintain this position for 30 seconds. Pay attention to breathing!
- Focus yourself on a mirror. Then oscillate to-and-fro, right-and-left, around your ankles keeping your pelvis still, according to breath rhythm hearing the air that enters and then exits from the lungs
- Repeat with eyes closed.
- Keep a little object and then lift it over your head and focus on it. With your extended arms move it with over and over wide circles maintaining focus on the object, according to the breath rhythm hearing the air that enter and then exits from the lungs
- Repeat with eyes closed. . Pay attention to breathing!
- Keep a little object and lift it over your head. Focus on it. Inhale. Then exhale and bend yourself forward taking the object on the floor. Wait 10 seconds and then inhaling lift again the object over your head. Pay attention to breathing!

2.3 Selection of the patients

Selection of the patients was based on a complete audiological, muscle-skeletal and stress balance (CAPPE questionnaire and PSQ).

The inclusion criteria are:

1. Acute or Chronic Tinnitus in alarm or resistance stress reaction phase: TRQ less than 80
2. CAPPE 's item "increasing with physical exercise" positive answer

3. PSQ score at least 15 as total score OR 4-5 score in "tension" sub-scale
4. Patient's tinnitus modulated by somatic manoeuvres as described by Levine et al. 2007
5. No tinnitus modulation t by Jendrassik manoeuvres. In our experience modulation by clenching, neck forceful flexion,... AND Jendrassik modulation means a no-specific facilitation of tinnitus perception to be distinguished from specific, treatable, somatic involvement
6. Trigger or tender point in the muscles specifically activated during forceful somatic manoeuvres, e.g masseter or anterior temporal regarding clenching, sterno-cleido-mastoideus regarding neck flexion or rotation, and so on

To determine individual Tinnitus specific reaction beside TRQ , Tinnitus Cognitive Questionnaire (TCQ) (Wilson &Henry 1998) was adopted. TCQ investigates patient approach to tinnitus with 13 negative (1-13) and 13 positive (14-26) thinking items, rated on a 0 - 4 point scale. For each item, respondents are asked to "indicate how often they have been aware of thinking a particular thought on occasions when they have noticed the tinnitus". The negative items are scored from 0 to 4 whereas the positive items are scored from 4 to 0. The total score is the sum of the scores of each item and ranges from 0 to 104. A high score represents a greater tendency to engage in negative cognitions in response to tinnitus and low engagement in positive cognitions.

TRQ, PSQ and TCQ represent the outcome measures of Tinnitus School Treatment. TRQ and PSQ are administered by the physician during selection/counselling while TCQ is administered by the physiotherapist at the first training session.

No specific drug was proposed but only those necessary for general health treatment (diabetes, hypertension,...) even through combined physical and pharmacological treatment has been proposed by Hahn et al. (2007).

Patients were controlled each month for 3 months and, successively, after six months, in order to modify home training exercises planning and to re-motivate them to therapy.

3. Conclusion

Tinnitus is a symptom that it is not possible to solve when it is chronic. Chronic disabling tinnitus is due to emotional-affective involvement induced by a pathological shift of patient attention to his/her tinnitus. Coping with tinnitus thus require a modification of the patient approach to inself perception through the modification of lifestyle, stressor removing, and diverting pathological attention. The aim of the tinnitus cure, generally speaking, is to reach a golden point in which patient is able to hear tinnitus but tinnitus is not disabling for the patient.

Tinnitus School is an educational approach aimed to help the patient to manage her/his symptom in order to restore a normal quality of life.

Tinnitus School, especially when it regards somatic subtype, requires both strict cooperation between the Physician and the Physiotherapist and as well that Physician is well trained in diagnosis and treatment of muscle-skeletal disturbances of head and neck.

According to the strict selection criteria adopted, we treated 24 patients, in 8 classes (6 males and 18 females, mean age 51,5 years old; TRQ 67 ± 7; TCQ 74 ± 6). No specific drugs were proposed. Regarding PSQ, mean total score was 17±2 and all the patients presented maximum tension sub-scale score.

All the patients were controlled each month for 3 months. In all of them tinnitus coping was referred to be good, with a positive increase of quality of life, documented by a decrease of

TRQ and TCQ scores, respectively to 38 ± 9 and 34 ± 4, as showed in fig.1.After six months, 18 patients were controlled (6 dropped out), but all maintained life-style modifications (sleep and diet regulation, regular physical exercise) with satisfying tinnitus coping.

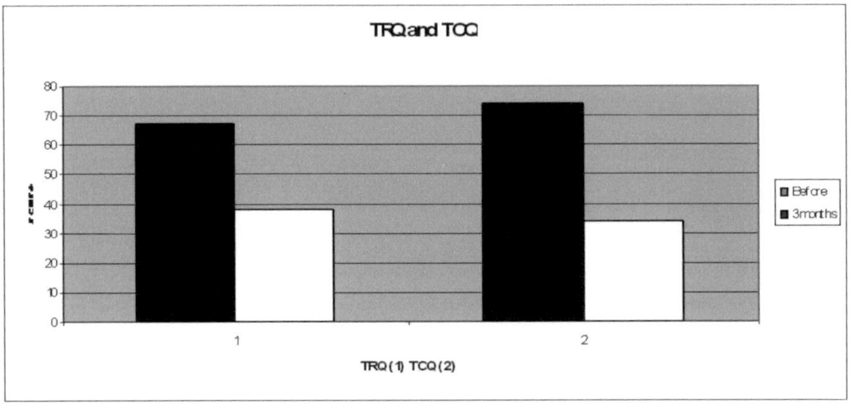

Fig. 1. TRQ and TCQ modifications after 3 months follow-up (mean values). Both reaction questionnaire and cognitive questionnaire scores are reduced, representing a positive increase of quality of life.

Follow-up2 PSQ re-scoring showed significant improvements for two of the stress scales and the overall score: After 10 sessions of training and three months of home training tinnitus patients showed a significant decrease of generally PSQ score, that to say generally perceived stress level, amelioration regards tension decrease (less positive answers) and joy increase (less negative answers), worries and demands remain unchanged, as already described by Weber et al. (2002). (Fig.2)

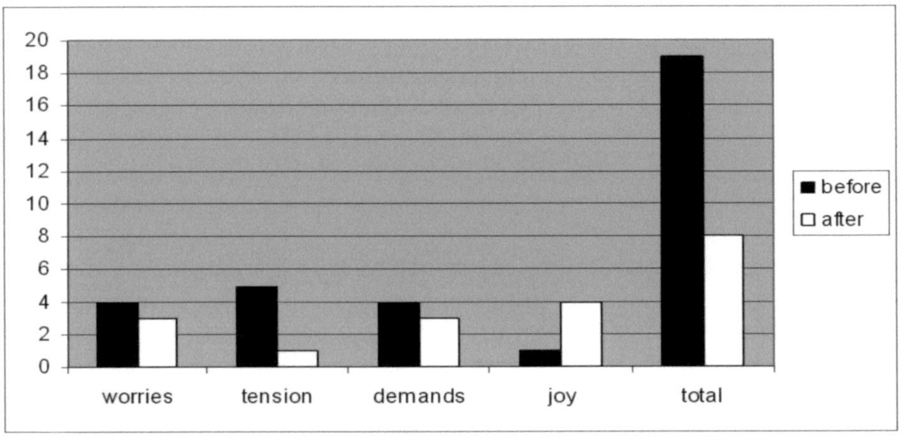

Fig. 2. PSQ mean subscales and total scores are showed (mean values). Scores regard pre-treatment and after 3-months follow-up. Worries and Demands subscales didn't n modify while tension and joy sub-scales ameliorated. Thus the total score is decreased after Tinnitus School program. Joy is presented in a reverse way with respect to the questionnaire in order to better represent the positive modifications.

Decreasing TCQ, TRQ and PSQ scores represent a significant improvement in the quality of life of the participants, suggesting therefore that educational approach could have an effect on the cognitive aspects of tinnitus and contributes positively to the management of tinnitus. Anyway, six month drop-out regarded 25% of the patients and this highlight how is difficult to maintain motivation to perform constantly home exercises.
Generally, evaluating the adopted psychometrics questionnaires, Tinnitus School program resulted in a significantly decrease of tinnitus disturbance (TRQ and TCQ) through a decreased perception of stress (PSQ) but it requires both a strict selection of the subjects and patients strongly motivated "to feel better"; furthermore adequate complete treatment of cervico-cephalic somatosensory disturbances is needed.
Further researches have to be pointed both to a better understanding of the basis of neurobiological connection between sound and motion and a better selection of somatic tinnitus sub-type patients. In fact, Tinnitus may represents a sort of auditory after-effect (Riecke et al 2011): an interrupted sound can be perceived as continuous when noise masks the interruption, creating an illusion of continuity. Recent findings have shown that adaptor sounds preceding an ambiguous target sound can influence the listeners' rating of target continuity. However, it remains unclear whether these aftereffects on perceived continuity influence sensory processes, decisional processes (i.e., criterion shifts), or both. It is reasonable to assume that somatic disturbances convey abnormal inputs on DCN creating something like spinal segmental sensitization described by Fisher (1997) to explain chronic myofascial pain. According to this idea, somatic inputs may represent the "sensorial noise" in the DCN that masks the interruption, creating an illusion of continuity, continuity that we know to be the prerequisite for inducing chronic Tinnitus at both cortical and limbic level.

4. Acknowledgment

We thanks Mrs Nayera Saad for checking the English translation; we are indebted with dott. Giampaolo De Sena that suggested to us spinal segmental sensitization model as a somatic tinnitus model and consequently with prof. Guido Brugnoni that introduced us in adopting Manual Medicine for somatic tinnitus diagnosis and treatment

5. References

Alpini, D. Cesarani, A. (2006) Tinnitus as an alarm bell: stress reaction tinnitus model. *ORL J Otorhinolaryngol Relat Spec.* Vol. 68(1), 31-6

Alpini, D. Cesarani, A. Hahn, A. (2007) Tinnitus school: an educational approach to tinnitus management based on a stress-reaction tinnitus model. *Int Tinnitus J.* Vol.13(1),63-68

Axelsson, A. Ringdahl, A. (1985) Tinnitus: a study of its prevalence and characteristics. *British J Audiol* Vol. 23. 53-62.

Bergado, JA. Lucas, M. Richter-Levin, G. (2011) Emotional tagging-A simple hypothesis in a complex reality. *Prog Neurobiol.* Vol.94(1).64-76

Biesinger, E. Kipman, U. Schatz, S. Langguth, B. (2010) Qigong for the treatment of tinnitus: a prospective randomized controlled study.*J psycosom Res* Vol. 69 (3). 299-304

Cluny, C. Norena, A. El Massioui, F, Chery-Croze, S. (2004) Reduced attention shift in response to auditory changes in subjects with tinnitus. *Audiol Neurootol* Vol.9. 294-202

Dehler, R. Dehler, F. Claussen, CF. Schneider, D. Just, E. (2000) Competitive-kinesthesic interaction therapy. *Int* Tinnitus J Vol. 6(1): 29-35

Dehmel, S .Cui, Y.L. Shore, S.E. (2008) Cross-modal interactions of auditory and somatic inputs in the brainstem and midbrain and their imbalance in tinnitus and deafness *Am J Audiol* Vol.17(2): 193–209

Feldman, H. Homolateral and contralateral masking of tinnitus by noise-bands and by pure tones. (1971) *Audiology* Vol.10(3):138–144.

Fliege, H. Rose, M. Arck, P. Walter ,O.B. Kocalevent,R.D., Weber, C. Klapp, B.F.The Perceived Stress Questionnaire (PSQ) reconsidered: validation and reference values from different clinical and healthy adult samples. (205) *Psychosom Med.* Vol.67(1):78-88

Fischer, A.A. (ed) Myofascial pain-Update in Diagnosis and Treatment. Phys Med Rehabil Clin North Am, Philadelphia, W.B. Saunders, 1997; p.153-169.

Hahn, A. Sejna, I,.Stolbova, K. Cocek, A. Combined laser-EGb 761 tinnitus therapy. (2001) *Acta Otolaryngol* Suppl.545:92-93.

Henry, J.L. Wilson, P.H. Tinnitus: a self-management guide for the ringing in your ears. Boston: Allyn and Bacon, 2001.

Horner, K.C. The emotional ear in stress. (2003) *Neusorscience Behav Rev* Vol.27: 437-446

Jousmäki and Hari (1998) Parchment-skin illusion: sound-biased touch. (1998) *Curr Biol.* Vol.12;8(6): 190-195

Kaltenbach, J.A. Tinnitus. Models and Mechanisms. (2010) *Hear Res* Vol.10(1):35-38

Levine, R.A Nam, E.C. Oron, Y. Melcher, J.R. Evidence for a Tinnitus subgroup responsive to somatosensory based treatment modalities. (2007) *Progress Brain Research* Vol 166: 195- 207

Malouff, J.J. Noble, W. Schutte, N.S Bhullar, N. The effectiveness of bibliotherapy in alleviating tinnitus-related distress (2010) *Journal of Psychosomatic Research* Vol.68 (2):245–251

Maigne, R. & Nieves, W.L. Diagnosis and Treatment of Pain of Vertebral Origin, Second Edition (Pain Management) Informa Healthcare - 568 pages, 2 edition 2005

Nodar, R.H. CAPPE - A strategy for counselling tinnitus patients. (1996) *Int Tinnitus J* Vol. 2(2): 111-114

Norena, A. J. An integrative model of tinnitus based on a central gain controlling neural sensitivity. (2010) *Neuroscience and Biobehavioral Reviews* Vol.10: 345-353

Rauschecker, J.P. Leaver, A.M. Muhlau, M. Tuning Out the Noise: Limbic-Auditory Interactions in Tinnitus. (2010) *Neuron* Vol.66, (24): 819-826

Renier, L.A. Anurova, I. De Volder, A. G. Carlson ,S . VanMeter, J. Multisensory Integration of Sounds and Vibrotactile Stimuli in Processing Stream for "What" and "Where". (2009) *The J. Neurosc.* Vol. 29(35): 10950-10960

Riecke, L. Micheyl, C. Vanbussel, M. Schreiner, C.S. Mendelsohn, D. Formisano, E. Recalibration of the auditory continuity illusion: Sensory and decisional effects. (2011) *Hear Res.* Vol. 27: 765-771.

Riga, M. Xenellis, J. Peraki, E. Ferekidou, E. Korres, S. Aural Symptomps in Patients with Tempero-Mandibular Joint Disorders. Multiple Frequency Tympanometry Provides Objective Evidence of Charges in Middle Ear Impedence. (2010) *Otol Neurotol* Vol. 31:456-461

Shulman, A. A final common pathway for tinnitus: the medial temporal lobe system. (1995) *Int Tinnitus J* Vol.1: 115-126

Shulman, A. Strashun, A.M. Goldstein, B.A. GABA-benzodiazepine-chloride receptor-targeted therapy for tinnitus control: preliminary report. (2002) *Int Tinnitus J.* Vol.8(1):30-38

Simmons, R. Dambra, C. Lobarinas, E. Stocking, C. Salvi, R. Head, Neck, and Eye Movements That Modulate Tinnitus. (2008) *Semin Hear.* Vol.29(4): 361–370.

Sindhusake, D. Golding, M. Wigney,D. Newall, P. Jakobsen, K. Mitchell, P. Factors predicting severity of tinnitus: a population-based assessment. (2004) *J Am Acad Audiol* Vol.15(4): 269-280.

Tavafian, S.S. Jamshidi, A. Mohammad, K. Montazeri, A. Low back pain education and short term quality of life: a randomized trial. (2007) *BMC Musculoskelet Disord.* Vol. 28;8:21

Tyler, R. Coelho, C. Tao, P. Ji, H. Gehringer, A. Gogel, S. Identifying Tinnitus Subgroups With Cluster Analysis (2008) *Am J Audiol.* Vol. 17(2): 176–184

Vanneste,S. Plazier, M. Van de Heyning, P. De Ridder, D. Transcutaneous electrical nerve stimulation (TENS) of upper cervical nerve (C2) for the treatment of somatic tinnitus (2010) *Exp Brain Res* Vol.204:283–287

Vanneste, S. Plazier, M. van der Loo, E. Van de Heyning, P. Congedo, M. De Ridder, D. The Neural Correlates of Tiinnitus-related distress. (2010) *Neuroimage* Vol.52: 470-480

Yang, Q. Vernet, M. Orssaud, C. Bonfils, P. Londero, A. Central Crosstalk for Somatic Tinnitus: Abnormal Vergence Eye Movements. (2010) *PLoS ONE* Vol.5(7): 11845-11852

Weber ,C. Arck, P. Mazurek, B. Klapp, B.F. Impact of a relaxation training on psychometric and immunologic parameters in tinnitus sufferers. (2002) *Psychosom Res.* Vol.52(1):29-33

Wilson, P.H. Henry, J. Bowen, M. Haralambous, G. Tinnitus reaction questionnaire: psychometric properties of a measure of distress associated with tinnitus. (1991) *J Speech Hearing Res* Vol.34: 197-201

Wilson, P.H. Henry, J. Tinnitus cognitions questionnaire: development and psychometric properties of a measure of dysfunctional cognitions associated with tinnitus. (1998) *Int Tinnitus J* Vol.4(1): 23-30.

Zenner, H.P. Zalaman, I.M. Cognitive tinnitus sensitization: Behavioural and neurophysiological aspects of tinnitus centralization. (2004) *Acta Otolaryngol* Vol. 124(4):436–439

Part 4

Tinnitus in the Emergency

5

Evaluation of Tinnitus in the Emergency Department

Kerry J. Welsh[1], Audrey R. Nath[1] and Matthew R. Lewin[2]
[1]*University of Texas Health Science Center at Houston*
[2]*California Academy of Sciences*
USA

1. Introduction

Tinnitus is defined as the perception of abnormal noise by the patient in the absence of an external acoustic source. It may be described as a ringing, whistling, buzzing, roaring, or clicking sound, although any type of sound may be reported. Tinnitus may be unilateral or bilateral, and can be described as occurring within the head or as a distant sound [1]. It may occur constantly or intermittently. Tinnitus severity may vary considerably, ranging from a minor annoyance for the patient to distressing enough for certain patients to consider suicide [2].

Tinnitus appears to be a very common symptom, with a reported prevalence ranging from 10 - 25 % [3,4]. Of the 35 - 50 million adults with this symptom, approximately 12 million visit a physician; 2 - 3 million of these patients are severely impacted by tinnitus [5]. Furthermore, these patients often have numerous associated comorbidities including anxiety, depression, and reduced general health [6-9]. Tinnitus occurs more frequently in Caucasians, men, and older age groups [10]. Other reported risk factors include exposure to loud noise, hearing loss, smoking, and hypertension [11,12]. Tinnitus has also been reported in approximately 36% of children, but often goes undocumented due to the infrequency of their spontaneously reporting it [13].

Numerous hypotheses have been developed for the pathophysiology of tinnitus; however, a precise mechanism has not been established [14]. Tinnitus may arise from any abnormality of the neural pathway from the cochlear neural axis to the auditory cortex. Proposed etiologies include damage to hair cells with accompanying excess stimulation of auditory nerves, increased activity in the auditory complex, and excessively active auditory nerves [3,15]. Multiple mechanisms likely account for tinnitus because of the complexity of the hearing pathways, and thus this symptom is non-specific.

Several classification types have been used to described tinnitus. One such method classifies tinnitus as objective or subjective. Objective tinnitus indicates that the sound may be heard by the physician by auscultation with a stethoscope over the head and neck adjacent to the patient's ear [3]. Subjective tinnitus is considerably more common, and is only perceived by the patient. This chapter will review the differential diagnosis of objective and subjective tinnitus as well as the evaluation and management of these patients.

2. Objective tinnitus

Objective tinnitus, occasionally referred to as somatosounds, is audible to the physician by use of a stethoscope or Doppler [15]. The tinnitus is often characterized by the patient as a clicking or pulsing sound. The cause is often due to a vascular abnormality, which may be arterial or venous in etiology [1]. Additional causes include neurologic lesions or eustachian tube dysfunction [15].

2.1 Vascular causes

i. Arterial sources. Arteriovenous shunts include both arteriovenous malformations and arteriovenous fistulas, and represent an important cause of tinnitus that is essential to recognize in the emergency department [1]. Congenital arteriovenous malformations are generally asymptomatic and are uncommon causes of tinnitus, whereas acquired arteriovenous shunts are more likely to be symptomatic. Approximately 10 -15 % of intracranial arteriovenous fistula are dural, but are more often responsible for tinnitus than neck or cerebral arteriovenous shunts [16]. Dural arteriovenous fistulas likely arise due to dural venous sinus thrombosis that is most often due to trauma, but may also be secondary to infections, neoplasms, or surgery [17]. Mortality from hemorrhage of a dural arteriovenous fistula ranges from 10 - 20% [17]; thus, appropriate diagnosis by emergency physicians is essential.

A second significant cause of acquired arteriovenous shunt that may cause tinnitus is a paraganglioma in the temporal bone, classified as either a glomus jugulare or glomus typanicum tumor [15]. Such tumors often cause the patient to perceive a constant blowing sound. Additional symptoms that may occur as the tumor enlarges include hearing loss, and deficits in cranial nerves VII - XII. These tumors are occasionally visualized as a vascular mass behind the tympanic membrane [15].

Rarely, tinnitus may be caused by dissecting aneurysms of the of the internal auditory canal or the vertebral artery [17]. Additional symptoms that may occur are pain, Horner's syndrome, cranial nerve deficits, subarachnoid hemorrhage, and transient ischemic attacks. Vasculopathies that predispose individuals to this condition include Marfan syndrome, osteogenesis imperfecta, and fibromuscular dysplasia [17].

Tinnitus may occasionally be the presenting symptom of atherosclerosis in the carotid artery [17,18]. The source of the somatosounds is stenosis in regions of the carotid artery that result in blood flow turbulence. Associated risk factors are those typical for atherosclerosis and include older age, smoking, diabetes, hyperlipidemia, and hypertension. Carotid bruits have been reported in patients with this source of tinnitus [18]. Tinnitus may also result from arterial bruits in other vessels in the temporal bone including branches of the external carotid, basilar, vertebral arteries, and vascular abnormalities located in the auditory canal [15,19]. These patients generally lack other otologic symptoms such as vertigo, hearing loss, otalgia, and symptoms of aural fullness [15].

ii. Venous sources. Tinnitus may also arise from venous sources. A venous origin of tinnitus may be differentiated from an arterial source by application of pressure on the ipsilateral jugular vein; this maneuver results in cessation of the tinnitus from venous sources [17].

The most important etiology of venous causes of tinnitus is pseudotumor cerebri, also called idiopathic intracranial hypertension. Pseudotumor cerebri classically occurs in young, obese, women. Pulsatile tinnitus in one series was reported to occur in 60% of patients;

accompanying symptoms include headache, visual disturbances, and retrobulbar pain [20]. Indeed, the combination of headache with pulsatile tinnitus is fairly specific for the diagnosis of pseudotumor cerebri [20-22]. The most common signs on physical exam include papilledema, loss of visual fields, and cranial nerve VI palsy. Occasionally, pseudotumor cerebri has been reported in the absence of papilledema [22-24]. Untreated pseudotumor cerebri may lead to permanent vision loss [25].

Venous hums are another source of tinnitus. They may be heard in patients with hypertension, which may be systemic or intracranial [15]. Another cause of venous hum tinnitus is a dehiscent jugular bulb, an aberrantly high location of the jugular bulb that extends into the middle ear space [15]. Dehiscent jugular bulb tinnitus results in a low-pitched, soft hum that decreases with activity, movement of the head, or application of jugular vein pressure. Hearing loss has been reported secondary to a dehiscent jugular bulb [26]. A dehiscent jugular bulb may be visualized behind the tympanic membrane, and must be differentiated from a glomus tumor [15].

2.2 Non-vascular causes

Palatal myoclonus and stapedial muscle spasm are two neurologic disorders that may cause objective tinnitus. Palatal myoclonus is caused by inappropriate contractions of the superior constrictor muscles, the salpingopharyngeus, the tensor veli palatini, and the levator veli palatini muscles [27]. The muscular contractions occur 10 - 240 times per minute, and occur intermittently; the objective tinnitus results from abrupt closure of the eustachian tube [28]. This condition may occur in any age group, and may be accompanied by temporomandibular joint pain or occipital headaches; other reported symptoms include hearing loss, alteration of sounds, and the sensation of aural pressure [15]. The diagnosis can be confirmed by viewing palatal myoclonic jerks or by listening with a Toynbee tube. This condition may occur secondary to other neurologic disorders such as cerebrovascular disease, central nervous system tumors, and multiple sclerosis [27].

Stapedial muscle spasm is an idiopathic condition that is described as a rumbling sensation in the ear [15]. It is often exacerbated by other noises such as speech. The diagnosis is made by visualizing contractions of the tympanic membrane that coincide with the sensation experienced by the patient. Stapedial muscle spasm is considered a benign, self-limited condition [15].

Finally, dysfunction of the eustachian tube may result in objective tinnitus [15]. This type of tinnitus is often described as a roaring sound that coincides with breathing. Patients may additionally report autophony and reverberation. The symptoms typically improve with lying down and recur after rising. It may be diagnosed by visualizing a fluttering of the tympanic membrane when the patient strongly inhales through the nose. This condition typically develops after a large weight loss of any type [15].

3. Subjective tinnitus

Subjective tinnitus refers to the perception of a sound that is not audible to the examiner. Patients describe the perceived sounds as a ringing, buzzing or clicking [29]. The causes for subjective tinnitus generally stem from hearing loss from damage to the auditory pathway anywhere from the external auditory canal to the auditory nerve.

External causes for subjective tinnitus include cerumen impaction as well as cerumen removal procedures [30], otitis externa [31] and temporomandibular disorders [32]. The presence of swelling in the external auditory canal may amplify tinnitus and must be ruled out with a thorough examination of the ears.

Within the middle ear, diseases of the ossicles may result in conductive hearing loss that results in a subjective tinnitus [33]. Patients with otosclerosis may describe a hearing loss which appears to improve in noisy environments. Otosclerosis may present in young or middle-aged adults and may be inherited in an autosomal dominant manner [34].

Damage to cochlear hair cells encompasses some of the most common causes of subjective tinnitus. Noise-induced hearing loss involves damage to cochlear hair cell from exposure to loud sounds in the environment, ranging from close proximity to explosions to overuse of headphones playing music at a high volume, and the severity of the tinnitus has been found to be associated with the degree of hearing loss [35]. These noise-induced insults may occur in children and young adults. In contrast, age-related hearing loss involves degeneration of cochlear hair cells, especially those in the higher frequency ranges, and may result in tinnitus corresponding to the frequencies of lost hearing [36].

Other components of the cochlea may be affected in addition to the hair cells that can result in hearing loss and subjective tinnitus. In Ménière's disease, there is an excessive accumulation of endolymph in the membranous labyrinth of the cochlea that leads to episodes of tinnitus, vertigo and progressive hearing loss [37]. Tinnitus in these subjects may vary over time, and reported handicap resulting from tinnitus has been found to associate with the stage of Ménière's disease [38].

Compression of the auditory nerve itself may result in increased firing of afferent neurons to the auditory cortex, leading to a gradual or abrupt onset of subjective tinnitus. Tumors within the internal auditory canal may lead to tinnitus and hearing loss [39,40]. Vestibular schwannomas, or acoustic neuromas, arise from the Schwann cells surrounding the eighth cranial nerve, resulting in both hearing loss and tinnitus as well as vertigo and disturbances in balance [41]. Patients with a strong suspicion for acoustic neuroma should undergo contrast-enhanced imaging to both make a diagnosis as well as to monitor the growth of the tumor, which tends to be slow [42]. The surgical resection of acoustic neuromas may also result in hearing loss and tinnitus from direct damage to the auditory nerve [43].

Involvement of the cerebral cortex and brainstem through tumors and infarctions may result in subjective tinnitus. Tumors of the inferior colliculus [44] and within the cerebellopontine angle [45] may cause tinnitus with auditory symptoms. Infarctions of the inferior colliculus [46], cerebellum [47], and the basal ganglia, thalamus and pons of the cerebral cortex [48] have been associated with subjective tinnitus.

There are a number of systemic illnesses that are known to cause subjective tinnitus. Anemia may result in a cerebral hypoxia that can cause symptoms of tinnitus, vertigo and headache, as in the setting of cancer-related anemia [49]. Hyperlipidemia may cause or worsen tinnitus, and lowering blood cholesterol levels has been found to improve subjective tinnitus [50]. Patients with low thyroid function may report some degree of hearing loss with tinnitus [51]. Multiple sclerosis may manifest with hearing impairment with tinnitus [52,53]. Syphilis may manifest in otologic symptoms in both early and late stages of the disease. The presence of otosyphilis may be characterized by hearing loss or hyperacusis with tinnitus along with vestibular disturbances [54].

Medications from nearly every major category may result in ototoxicity and tinnitus. The use of salicylates, such as aspirin, may result in damage to the cochlea spiral ganglion neurons [55] and changes in cochlear NMDA receptor currents [56]. Aminoglycoside antibiotics, such as gentamicin, are well known to cause hearing loss and vestibular damage [57]. Loop diuretics, such as furosemide, may result in transient or permanent ototoxicity, and these effects may be minimized by delivery with slow infusion rather than bolus injection or using divided oral doses [58]. Additionally, many chemotherapeutic agents [59], heavy metals [60,61] and anti-malarial drugs [62,63] may contribute to hearing loss and tinnitus.

Finally, psychiatric stressors may worsen the handicap resulting from subjective tinnitus. Depression [64] and fibromyalgia [65] have been found to associate with and exacerbate chronic tinnitus. It should be noted that subjective tinnitus generally differs from auditory hallucinations observed in psychotic disorders by the nature of the perceived sound; tinnitus generally manifests as a more simple ringing or humming, whereas auditory hallucinations tend to involve more complex sounds or speech [66].

4. Diagnostic evaluation of tinnitus

The main goal of the evaluation of tinnitus in the emergency department is to identify life-threatening causes, preserve hearing, identify causes that are treatable, and provide the appropriate referral and symptomatic treatment. The initial evaluation of tinnitus begins with a complete history, including the onset, location, characteristics, associated symptoms, pattern, alleviating/exacerbating factors, past medical history and surgeries, and medication use. The onset of tinnitus should be characterized as sudden versus gradual. A sudden onset of tinnitus is concerning, and may indicate a vascular or traumatic etiology. Questions regarding the pattern of tinnitus should attempt to differentiate pulsatile from continuous or episodic tinnitus. Pulsatile tinnitus is frequently due to a vascular source whereas Ménière's disease tends to be episodic. Specific associated symptoms to inquire about include hearing loss, vertigo, and aural fullness. The impact of patient positioning on the tinnitus should be asked; specifically, eustachian tube dysfunction is often alleviated by lying down. A past medical history of hyperlipidemia or diabetes may indicate carotid artery atherosclerosis, whereas a thyroid disorder or anemia may suggest a high output cause. Finally, a number of medications are known to cause tinnitus.

A thorough head and neck exam should be performed on all patients presenting with tinnitus. A search for an objective source of tinnitus should be performed by auscultation of the auricular region, the mastoid, and the carotid arteries. Objective tinnitus secondary to a venous etiology is identified by disappearance of the sound when the ipsilateral jugular vein is compressed. Careful otoscopy should be performed to evaluate for middle-ear infection, cerumen impaction, a dehiscent jugular bulb, or glomus tumor. The oral cavity should be examined for contractions of the palatal muscles. The cranial nerves should be evaluated for evidence of hearing loss or brainstem dysfunction. Finally, a fundoscopic exam should be performed to look for papilledema in suspected cases of pseudotumor cerebri.

Diagnostic testing should be guided by the results of the history and physical examination. A complete blood count and thyroid function tests may reveal conditions that cause increased cardiac output and cerebral blood flow that can result in tinnitus. Contrast enhanced computed tomography (CT) should be performed on patients with a tympanic mass visible on otoscopy, which may reveal jugular bulb abnormalities, glomus tumors, and vascular abnormalities. CT or MR angiography may be needed to diagnose dissecting aneurysms and arteriovenous fistulas. Carotid ultrasonography may confirm suspected carotid atherosclerotic artery disease. A lumbar puncture should be performed in patients who are being considered for a diagnosis of pseudotumor cerebri. The suggested approach to patients with tinnitus is depicted in Figures 1 and 2.

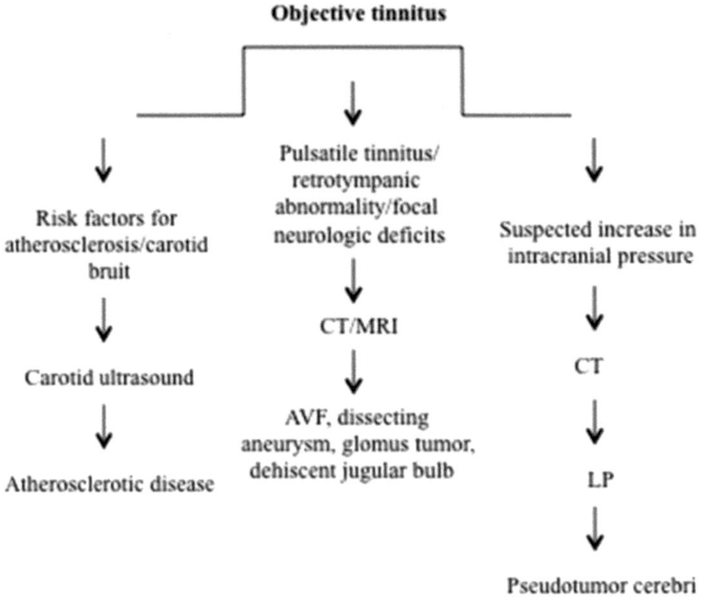

Fig. 1. Suggested approach to objective tinnitus in the emergency department.

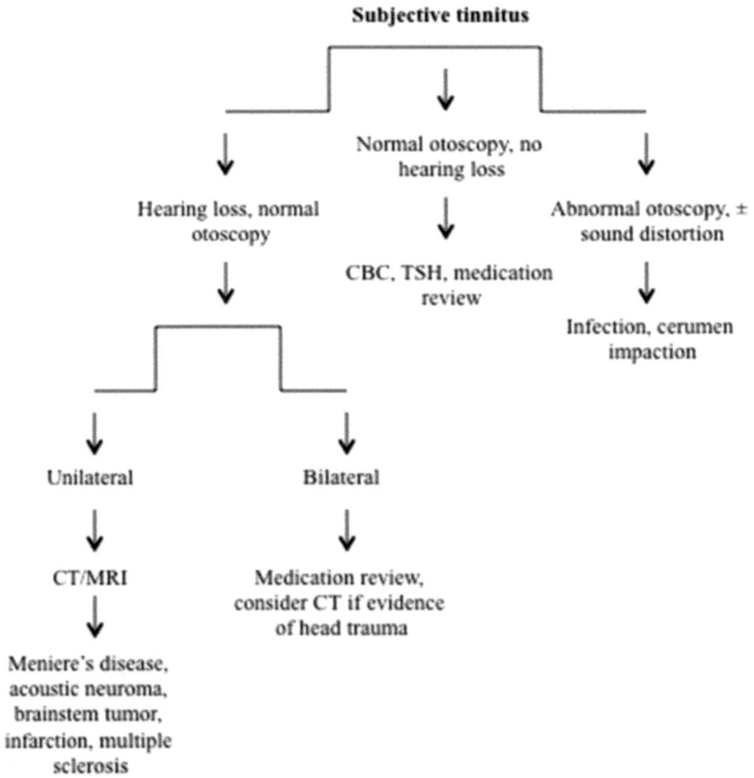

Fig. 2. Suggested approach to subjective tinnitus in the emergency department.

5. Management

The management of tinnitus first involves treating identified underlying causes. Tinnitus secondary to ototoxic medications may resolve after discontinuing the medication. Patients with arteriovenous fistula or dehiscent jugular bulb may be treated with vessel ligation or embolization. Those with glomus tumors can be referred for surgical resection or angiographic embolization. Carotid endarterectomy may benefit patients with tinnitus secondary to carotid artery atherosclerosis if the carotid artery stenosis is greater than 60% [67-69]. Patients with benign venous hums or arterial bruits may simply need reassurance, but may be referred for surgical ligation of the vessel if the tinnitus causes significant reduction in quality of life.

Patients with pseudotumor cerebri require intense follow-up with neurology and ophthalmology [70]. While lumbar punctures provide temporary relief, the benefit is short-term due to the rapid reformation of CSF and is not recommend as the primary therapy because of potential complications. Medical management involves treatment with carbonic anhydrase inhibitors, specifically acetazolamide at starting at doses of 500 mg twice daily [71]. Loop diuretics such as furosemide (20 - 40 mg/day in adults) are an adjunctive therapy [72]. Weight reduction also improves symptoms and is a critical component of management [73-75].

Patients with palatal myoclonus or eustachian tube dysfunction should be referred to an otolaryngologist for management. Injection of botulinum toxin into the palate has been successful for patients with tinnitus secondary to palatal muscle myoclonus [76]. Eustachian tube dysfunction may be managed by treatment with mucosal irritants such as tetracycline to the nose that cause disruption of the orifice of the eustachian tube [15]; alternatively, the nasopharyngeal orifice may be surgically closed [77] or silicone plugs placed through the middle ear [78].

Unfortunately, there are very few effective treatments specifically for tinnitus. Gabapentin resulted in a significant improvement in tinnitus annoyance scores for patients with tinnitus secondary to trauma [79], but does not appear to be effective in relieving idiopathic tinnitus [79,80]. Alprazolam was reported to decrease the loudness of tinnitus in one trial [81], whereas a more recent study failed to find an effect on tinnitus loudness or the Tinnitus Handicap Inventory [82]. Clinical trials of the tricyclic antidepressant nortriptyline significantly reduced tinnitus, depression, and the resulting disability [83,84]. However, caution should be used with prescribing these drugs in the emergency department due to the dangers of overdose in suicidal patients.

Many experimental therapies warrant consideration in patients with tinnitus unresponsive to medications. The use of repetitive transcranial magnetic stimulation (rTMS) to stimulate regions in and around temporal auditory cortex has had some success in cases of chronic tinnitus [85-87]. Finally, behavioral based therapies such as tinnitus retraining therapy, masking devices, and biofeedback therapy have reported success [10,88]; consideration should be given to referring patients to providers who can provide these interventions.

6. References

[1] Liyanage SH, Singh A, Savundra P, Kalan A. Pulsatile tinnitus. The Journal of laryngology and otology. 2006 Feb;120(2):93-7.

[2] Lewis JE, Stephens SD, McKenna L. Tinnitus and suicide. Clinical otolaryngology and allied sciences. 1994 Feb;19(1):50-4.

[3] Crummer RW, Hassan GA. Diagnostic approach to tinnitus. American family physician. 2004 Jan 1;69(1):120-6.

[4] Shargorodsky J, Curhan GC, Farwell WR. Prevalence and characteristics of tinnitus among US adults. The American journal of medicine. 2010 Aug;123(8):711-8.

[5] Adams PF, Hendershot GE, Marano MA. Current estimates from the National Health Interview Survey, 1996. Vital and health statistics Series 10, Data from the National Health Survey. 1999 Oct(200):1-203.

[6] Crocetti A, Forti S, Ambrosetti U, Bo LD. Questionnaires to evaluate anxiety and depressive levels in tinnitus patients. Otolaryngology--head and neck surgery : official journal of American Academy of Otolaryngology-Head and Neck Surgery. 2009 Mar;140(3):403-5.

[7] Folmer RL, Griest SE, Meikle MB, Martin WH. Tinnitus severity, loudness, and depression. Otolaryngology--head and neck surgery : official journal of American Academy of Otolaryngology-Head and Neck Surgery. 1999 Jul;121(1):48-51.

[8] Schleuning AJ, 2nd. Management of the patient with tinnitus. The Medical clinics of North America. 1991 Nov;75(6):1225-37.

[9] Tyler RS, Baker LJ. Difficulties experienced by tinnitus sufferers. The Journal of speech and hearing disorders. 1983 May;48(2):150-4.

[10] Lockwood AH, Salvi RJ, Burkard RF. Tinnitus. The New England journal of medicine. 2002 Sep 19;347(12):904-10.

[11] Axelsson A, Ringdahl A. Tinnitus--a study of its prevalence and characteristics. British journal of audiology. 1989 Feb;23(1):53-62.

[12] Nondahl DM, Cruickshanks KJ, Wiley TL, Klein R, Klein BE, Tweed TS. Prevalence and 5-year incidence of tinnitus among older adults: the epidemiology of hearing loss study. Journal of the American Academy of Audiology. 2002 Jun;13(6):323-31.

[13] Shetye A, Kennedy V. Tinnitus in children: an uncommon symptom? Archives of disease in childhood. 2010 Aug;95(8):645-8.

[14] Seidman MD, Standring RT, Dornhoffer JL. Tinnitus: current understanding and contemporary management. Current opinion in otolaryngology & head and neck surgery. 2010 Oct;18(5):363-8.

[15] Fortune DS, Haynes DS, Hall JW, 3rd. Tinnitus. Current evaluation and management. The Medical clinics of North America. 1999 Jan;83(1):153-62, x.

[16] Madani G, Connor SE. Imaging in pulsatile tinnitus. Clinical radiology. 2009 Mar;64(3):319-28.

[17] Sismanis A. Pulsatile tinnitus. Otolaryngologic clinics of North America. 2003 Apr;36(2):389-402, viii.

[18] Sismanis A, Stamm MA, Sobel M. Objective tinnitus in patients with atherosclerotic carotid artery disease. The American journal of otology. 1994 May;15(3):404-7.

[19] Herzog JA, Bailey S, Meyer J. Vascular loops of the internal auditory canal: a diagnostic dilemma. The American journal of otology. 1997 Jan;18(1):26-31.

[20] Wall M, George D. Idiopathic intracranial hypertension. A prospective study of 50 patients. Brain : a journal of neurology. 1991 Feb;114 (Pt 1A):155-80.

[21] Rudnick E, Sismanis A. Pulsatile tinnitus and spontaneous cerebrospinal fluid rhinorrhea: indicators of benign intracranial hypertension syndrome. Otology & neurotology : official publication of the American Otological Society, American

Neurotology Society [and] European Academy of Otology and Neurotology. 2005 Mar;26(2):166-8.

[22] Wang SJ, Silberstein SD, Patterson S, Young WB. Idiopathic intracranial hypertension without papilledema: a case-control study in a headache center. Neurology. 1998 Jul;51(1):245-9.

[23] Mathew NT, Ravishankar K, Sanin LC. Coexistence of migraine and idiopathic intracranial hypertension without papilledema. Neurology. 1996 May;46(5):1226-30.

[24] Quattrone A, Bono F, Fera F, Lavano A. Isolated unilateral abducens palsy in idiopathic intracranial hypertension without papilledema. European journal of neurology : the official journal of the European Federation of Neurological Societies. 2006 Jun;13(6):670-1.

[25] Corbett JJ, Savino PJ, Thompson HS, et al. Visual loss in pseudotumor cerebri. Follow-up of 57 patients from five to 41 years and a profile of 14 patients with permanent severe visual loss. Archives of neurology. 1982 Aug;39(8):461-74.

[26] Haupert MS, Madgy DN, Belenky WM, Becker JW. Unilateral conductive hearing loss secondary to a high jugular bulb in a pediatric patient. Ear, nose, & throat journal. 1997 Jul;76(7):468-9.

[27] Seidman MD, Arenberg JG, Shirwany NA. Palatal myoclonus as a cause of objective tinnitus: a report of six cases and a review of the literature. Ear, nose, & throat journal. 1999 Apr;78(4):292-4, 6-7.

[28] Slack RW, Soucek SO, Wong K. Sonotubometry in the investigation of objective tinnitus and palatal myoclonus: a demonstration of eustachian tube opening. The Journal of laryngology and otology. 1986 May;100(5):529-31.

[29] Hall III JW, Haynes DS. Audiologic assessment and consultation of the tinnitus patient. Semin Hear. 2001;22:37-50.

[30] Folmer RL, Shi BY. Chronic tinnitus resulting from cerumen removal procedures. Int Tinnitus J. 2004;10(1):42-6.

[31] Kurnatowski P, Filipiak J. Otitis externa: the analysis of relationship between particular signs/symptoms and species and genera of identified microorganisms. Wiad Parazytol. 2008;54(1):37-41.

[32] Bernhardt O, Mundt T, Welk A, et al. Signs and symptoms of temporomandibular disorders and the incidence of tinnitus. J Oral Rehabil. 2011 Apr 23.

[33] Deggouj N, Castelein S, Gerard JM, Decat M, Gersdorff M. Tinnitus and otosclerosis. B-ENT. 2009;5(4):241-4.

[34] Ealy M, Smith RJ. Otosclerosis. Adv Otorhinolaryngol. 2011;70:122-9.

[35] Mazurek B, Olze H, Haupt H, Szczepek AJ. The more the worse: the grade of noise-induced hearing loss associates with the severity of tinnitus. Int J Environ Res Public Health. 2010 Aug;7(8):3071-9.

[36] Nicolas-Puel C, Faulconbridge RL, Guitton M, Puel JL, Mondain M, Uziel A. Characteristics of tinnitus and etiology of associated hearing loss: a study of 123 patients. Int Tinnitus J. 2002;8(1):37-44.

[37] Semaan MT, Megerian CA. Meniere's disease: a challenging and relentless disorder. Otolaryngol Clin North Am. 2011 Apr;44(2):383-403, ix.

[38] Sanchez RI, Perez Garrigues H, Rodriguez Rivera V. Clinical characteristics of tinnitus in Meniere's disease. Acta Otorrinolaringol Esp. 2010;61(5):327-31.

[39] Ishikawa T, Kawamata T, Kawashima A, et al. Meningioma of the internal auditory canal with rapidly progressive hearing loss: case report. Neurol Med Chir (Tokyo). 2011;51(3):233-5.
[40] Wuertenberger CJ, Rosahl SK. Vertigo and tinnitus caused by vascular compression of the vestibulocochlear nerve, not intracanalicular vestibular schwannoma: review and case presentation. Skull Base. 2009 Nov;19(6):417-24.
[41] Agrawal Y, Clark JH, Limb CJ, Niparko JK, Francis HW. Predictors of vestibular schwannoma growth and clinical implications. Otol Neurotol. 2010 Jul;31(5):807-12.
[42] Sriskandan N, Connor SE. The role of radiology in the diagnosis and management of vestibular schwannoma. Clin Radiol. 2011 Apr;66(4):357-65.
[43] Cope TE, Baguley DM, Moore BC. Tinnitus Loudness in Quiet and Noise After Resection of Vestibular Schwannoma. Otol Neurotol. 2011 Jan 8.
[44] Missori P, Delfini R, Cantore G. Tinnitus and hearing loss in pineal region tumours. Acta Neurochir (Wien). 1995;135(3-4):154-8.
[45] Hodges TR, Karikari IO, Nimjee SM, Tibaleka J, Cummings TJ, Friedman AH. Calcifying Pseudoneoplasm of the Cerebellopontine Angle: Case Report. Neurosurgery. 2011 Mar 15.
[46] Choi SY, Song JJ, Hwang JM, Kim JS. Tinnitus in fourth nerve palsy: an indicator for an intra-axial lesion. J Neuroophthalmol. 2010 Dec;30(4):325-7.
[47] Martines F, Dispenza F, Gagliardo C, Martines E, Bentivegna D. Sudden sensorineural hearing loss as prodromal symptom of anterior inferior cerebellar artery infarction. ORL J Otorhinolaryngol Relat Spec. 2011;73(3):137-40.
[48] Sugiura S, Uchida Y, Nakashima T, Yoshioka M, Ando F, Shimokata H. Tinnitus and brain MRI findings in Japanese elderly. Acta Otolaryngol. 2008 May;128(5):525-9.
[49] Cunningham RS. Anemia in the oncology patient: cognitive function and cancer. Cancer Nurs. 2003 Dec;26(6 Suppl):38S-42S.
[50] Olzowy B, Canis M, Hempel JM, Mazurek B, Suckfull M. Effect of atorvastatin on progression of sensorineural hearing loss and tinnitus in the elderly: results of a prospective, randomized, double-blind clinical trial. Otol Neurotol. 2007 Jun;28(4):455-8.
[51] Bhatia PL, Gupta OP, Agrawal MK, Mishr SK. Audiological and vestibular function tests in hypothyroidism. Laryngoscope. 1977 Dec;87(12):2082-9.
[52] Nishida H, Tanaka Y, Okada M, Inoue Y. Evoked otoacoustic emissions and electrocochleography in a patient with multiple sclerosis. Ann Otol Rhinol Laryngol. 1995 Jun;104(6):456-62.
[53] Rodriguez-Casero MV, Mandelstam S, Kornberg AJ, Berkowitz RG. Acute tinnitus and hearing loss as the initial symptom of multiple sclerosis in a child. Int J Pediatr Otorhinolaryngol. 2005 Jan;69(1):123-6.
[54] Yimtae K, Srirompotong S, Lertsukprasert K. Otosyphilis: a review of 85 cases. Otolaryngol Head Neck Surg. 2007 Jan;136(1):67-71.
[55] Wei L, Ding D, Salvi R. Salicylate-induced degeneration of cochlea spiral ganglion neurons-apoptosis signaling. Neuroscience. 2010 Jun 16;168(1):288-99.
[56] Puel JL. Cochlear NMDA receptor blockade prevents salicylate-induced tinnitus. B-ENT. 2007;3 Suppl 7:19-22.
[57] Xie J, Talaska AE, Schacht J. New developments in aminoglycoside therapy and ototoxicity. Hear Res. 2011 May 27.

[58] Rybak LP. Pathophysiology of furosemide ototoxicity. J Otolaryngol. 1982 Apr;11(2):127-33.
[59] Dille MF, Konrad-Martin D, Gallun F, et al. Tinnitus onset rates from chemotherapeutic agents and ototoxic antibiotics: results of a large prospective study. J Am Acad Audiol. 2010 Jun;21(6):409-17.
[60] Arda HN, Tuncel U, Akdogan O, Ozluoglu LN. The role of zinc in the treatment of tinnitus. Otol Neurotol. 2003 Jan;24(1):86-9.
[61] Kim SJ, Jeong HJ, Myung NY, et al. The protective mechanism of antioxidants in cadmium-induced ototoxicity in vitro and in vivo. Environ Health Perspect. 2008 Jul;116(7):854-62.
[62] Ralli M, Lobarinas E, Fetoni AR, Stolzberg D, Paludetti G, Salvi R. Comparison of salicylate- and quinine-induced tinnitus in rats: development, time course, and evaluation of audiologic correlates. Otol Neurotol. 2010 Jul;31(5):823-31.
[63] Bortoli R, Santiago M. Chloroquine ototoxicity. Clin Rheumatol. 2007 Nov;26(11):1809-10.
[64] Langguth B, Landgrebe M, Kleinjung T, Sand GP, Hajak G. Tinnitus and depression. World J Biol Psychiatry. 2011 May 13.
[65] Waylonis GW, Heck W. Fibromyalgia syndrome. New associations. Am J Phys Med Rehabil. 1992 Dec;71(6):343-8.
[66] Shergill SS, Brammer MJ, Fukuda R, Williams SC, Murray RM, McGuire PK. Engagement of brain areas implicated in processing inner speech in people with auditory hallucinations. Br J Psychiatry. 2003 Jun;182:525-31.
[67] Endarterectomy for asymptomatic carotid artery stenosis. Executive Committee for the Asymptomatic Carotid Atherosclerosis Study. JAMA : the journal of the American Medical Association. 1995 May 10;273(18):1421-8.
[68] Halliday A, Mansfield A, Marro J, et al. Prevention of disabling and fatal strokes by successful carotid endarterectomy in patients without recent neurological symptoms: randomised controlled trial. Lancet. 2004 May 8;363(9420):1491-502.
[69] Hobson RW, 2nd, Weiss DG, Fields WS, et al. Efficacy of carotid endarterectomy for asymptomatic carotid stenosis. The Veterans Affairs Cooperative Study Group. The New England journal of medicine. 1993 Jan 28;328(4):221-7.
[70] Wall M. Sensory visual testing in idiopathic intracranial hypertension: measures sensitive to change. Neurology. 1990 Dec;40(12):1859-64.
[71] Kesler A, Hadayer A, Goldhammer Y, Almog Y, Korczyn AD. Idiopathic intracranial hypertension: risk of recurrences. Neurology. 2004 Nov 9;63(9):1737-9.
[72] Lee AG, Anderson R, Kardon RH, Wall M. Presumed "sulfa allergy" in patients with intracranial hypertension treated with acetazolamide or furosemide: cross-reactivity, myth or reality? American journal of ophthalmology. 2004 Jul;138(1):114-8.
[73] Newborg B. Pseudotumor cerebri treated by rice reduction diet. Archives of internal medicine. 1974 May;133(5):802-7.
[74] Kupersmith MJ, Gamell L, Turbin R, Peck V, Spiegel P, Wall M. Effects of weight loss on the course of idiopathic intracranial hypertension in women. Neurology. 1998 Apr;50(4):1094-8.

[75] Johnson LN, Krohel GB, Madsen RW, March GA, Jr. The role of weight loss and acetazolamide in the treatment of idiopathic intracranial hypertension (pseudotumor cerebri). Ophthalmology. 1998 Dec;105(12):2313-7.
[76] Bryce GE, Morrison MD. Botulinum toxin treatment of essential palatal myoclonus tinnitus. The Journal of otolaryngology. 1998 Aug;27(4):213-6.
[77] Orlandi RR, Shelton C. Endoscopic closure of the eustachian tube. American journal of rhinology. 2004 Nov-Dec;18(6):363-5.
[78] Sato T, Kawase T, Yano H, Suetake M, Kobayashi T. Trans-tympanic silicone plug insertion for chronic patulous Eustachian tube. Acta oto-laryngologica. 2005 Nov;125(11):1158-63.
[79] Bauer CA, Brozoski TJ. Effect of gabapentin on the sensation and impact of tinnitus. The Laryngoscope. 2006 May;116(5):675-81.
[80] Piccirillo JF, Finnell J, Vlahiotis A, Chole RA, Spitznagel E, Jr. Relief of idiopathic subjective tinnitus: is gabapentin effective? Archives of otolaryngology--head & neck surgery. 2007 Apr;133(4):390-7.
[81] Johnson RM, Brummett R, Schleuning A. Use of alprazolam for relief of tinnitus. A double-blind study. Archives of otolaryngology--head & neck surgery. 1993 Aug;119(8):842-5.
[82] Jalali MM, Kousha A, Naghavi SE, Soleimani R, Banan R. The effects of alprazolam on tinnitus: a cross-over randomized clinical trial. Medical science monitor : international medical journal of experimental and clinical research. 2009 Nov;15(11):PI55-60.
[83] Sullivan M, Katon W, Russo J, Dobie R, Sakai C. A randomized trial of nortriptyline for severe chronic tinnitus. Effects on depression, disability, and tinnitus symptoms. Archives of internal medicine. 1993 Oct 11;153(19):2251-9.
[84] Dobie RA, Sakai CS, Sullivan MD, Katon WJ, Russo J. Antidepressant treatment of tinnitus patients: report of a randomized clinical trial and clinical prediction of benefit. The American journal of otology. 1993 Jan;14(1):18-23.
[85] De Ridder D. Should rTMS for tinnitus be performed left-sided, ipsilaterally or contralaterally, and is it a treatment or merely investigational? Eur J Neurol. 2010 Jul;17(7):891-2.
[86] Meeus OM, De Ridder D, Van de Heyning PH. Transcranial magnetic stimulation (TMS) in tinnitus patients. B-ENT. 2009;5(2):89-100.
[87] Khedr EM, Rothwell JC, El-Atar A. One-year follow up of patients with chronic tinnitus treated with left temporoparietal rTMS. Eur J Neurol. 2009 Mar;16(3):404-8.
[88] Andersson G, Lyttkens L. A meta-analytic review of psychological treatments for tinnitus. British journal of audiology. 1999 Aug;33(4):201-10.

Part 5

Tinnitus and Noise Induced Hearing Loss

6

Medico-Legal Decision Making in NIHL-Related Tinnitus

P.H. Dejonckere
Federal Institute of Occupational Diseases, Brussels,
Dept. of Neurosciences, Katholieke Universiteit Leuven,
Belgium

1. Introduction

In clinical practice, tinnitus is a quite common symptom in patients with chronic acoustic trauma, and noise-induced hearing loss (NIHL). A review of the current state of knowledge on tinnitus in relation to noise exposure and hearing loss has been recently (Poole, 2010) published by the UK Health & Safety Executive. 252 publications were reviewed. The prevalence of tinnitus in populations exposed to noise at work is reported to be between 5,9% and 87,5%. Factors such as the type of subjects (e.g. health surveillance, compensation claimant), the characteristics of the noise exposure and the definition of tinnitus used apparently contribute to this variability. Several publications have shown that the prevalence of tinnitus in workers exposed to noise at work is significantly higher than in non-exposed workers. The majority of the published papers support the idea that there is an association between tinnitus and noise-induced hearing loss: the prevalence of tinnitus in workers with NIHL appears to be higher, and the workers with tinnitus have more severe NIHL.

In a medico-legal context, tinnitus is mostly a subsidiary item of claim, additional to that for noise-induced hearing loss. However, tinnitus may also be the principal or only complaint, e.g. in patients with a specific and selective noise-induced dip on 4 KHz but without obvious repercussion on their social hearing. Further, as in some cases tinnitus may cause devastating (and objectivable) effects on lifestyle and ability to work, it may attract higher levels of compensation than hearing loss (Coles, 2000).

In such a medico-legal situation, when e.g. the patient claims compensation for an occupational disease, potential financial advantage may be a strong motivation for feigning or exaggeration. The essentially subjective nature of tinnitus renders it very difficult to make – at least in some patients - equitable medico-legal decision about presence and severity of tinnitus. This implies that assessment needs to involve a large set of parameters, combining subjective with objective items (Nieschalk & Stoll, 2002).

The proposed method for medicolegally evaluating tinnitus in context of NIHL is based on a rational, echeloned progression in decision making: at each step, a quite large number of elementary (cellular) decisions, easy to make and reproducible among different experts, leads to the higher decision level. Four of such levels are worked out and formulated, with respectively 65, 12, 4 and 1 decisions. The final decision is then: accept or reject the tinnitus as a true component of the occupational disorder (noise-induced cochlear damage).

Directly related to this decision is the determination of the % of disability / impairment which may be attributed for this tinnitus component. The main purposes are to reach an optimal consistency among experts in these decisions, and to offer optimal transparency in case of litigation. The final aim is maximal equity.
However, the proposed system is not intended for being more than a methodological support. Adequate decision making, even at elementary level, requires from the expert / evaluator an exhaustive and encyclopedic knowledge of otoneurology.

2. The decision making system

(Dejonckere & Lebacq, 2005)

The four decision levels are structured as follows (Fig. 1):

Level 4

4.1.Final decision: Accept or reject.
4.2.If tinnitus is accepted, how much % impairment / invalidity ?

Level 3 (4 decisions)

3.1.Is the patient reliable ?
3.2.Besides the tinnitus, does the patient also demonstrate an occupational hearing loss ?
3.3.Is there a link between tinnitus and occupational hearing loss ?
3.4.Is the tinnitus disabilitating, and if so, to what extent ?
A positive decision about all four of these essential aspects is requested for acknowledging the tinnitus as a part of the occupational disease, and providing compensation.

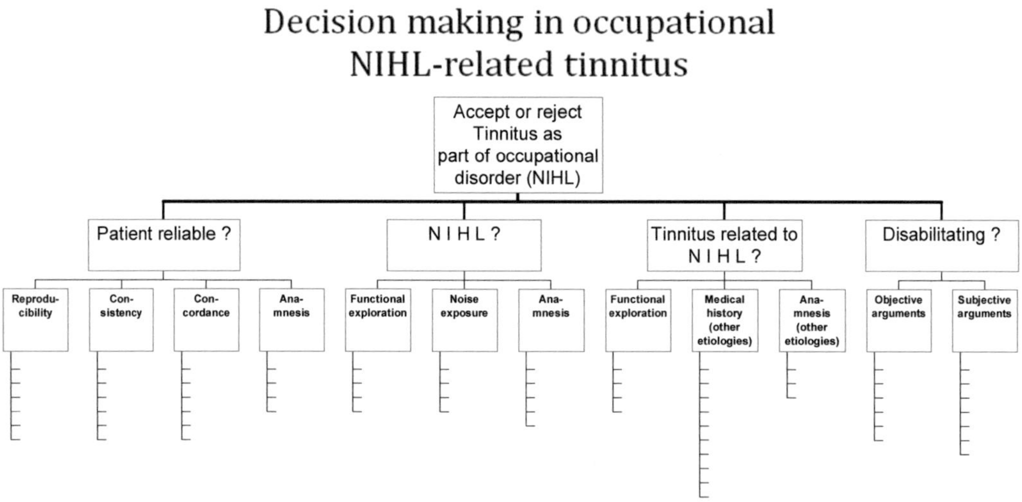

Fig. 1. Diagram showing the 4 levels of decision making, with respectively 65, 12, 4 and 1 decisions.

Level 2 (12 decisions)

As a general rule, possible answers are:

"Affirmative": in agreement, evident, compatible, plausible, concordant.

"Neutral": dubious, only partially in agreement, unclear, non evident, or non relevant item, or information lacking.
"Negative": not in agreement, incompatible, discordant, irrealistic, unacceptable.

In case of one or more "non-affirmative" responses, the expert needs to make a weighing in order to come to a final positive or negative decision for each question of the level 3.

Decisions at level 2 pertaining to 3.1. Is the patient reliable ?

2.1.Are measurements based on patient's responses reproducible ?
2.2.Are different approaches of a same physiological phenomenon consistent ?
2.3.Are subjective data concordant with objective data ?
2.4.Are the anamnestic data compatible with the (psycho-)physiological data ?

Decisions at level 2 pertaining to 3.2.: Besides the tinnitus, does the patient also demonstrate an occupational hearing loss ?

2.5. Does the hearing loss show the characteristics of NIHL at functional hearing assessment ?
2.6. Has the patient actually been exposed to harmful occupational noise ?
2.7. Is the anamnesis and is the history of complaints suggestive for progressive occupational hearing loss ?

Decisions at level 2 pertaining to 3.3.: Is there a link between tinnitus and occupational hearing loss ?

2.8. Does the functional assessment of tinnitus (tinnitometry) suggest the etiology of cochlear noise damage ?
2.9. Does the medical history demonstrate compatibility of tinnitus with the etiology of cochlear noise damage ?
2.10. Is the anamnesis and is the history of complaints suggestive for tinnitus related to progressive occupational hearing loss ?

Decisions at level 2 pertaining to 3.4.: Is the tinnitus disabilitating, and if so, to what extent ?

2.11. Are there convincing objective elements ?
2.12. Are there convincing subjective elements ?

Level 1 (65 decisions)

As a general rule, as for level 2, the possible answers are:

"Affirmative": in agreement, evident, compatible, plausible, concordant.
"Neutral": dubious, only partially in agreement, unclear, non evident, or non relevant item, or information lacking
"Negative": not in agreement, incompatible, discordant, irrealistic, unacceptable.

Ad 2.1. Are measurements based on patient's responses reproducible ?

Reproducibility of psycho-acoustic data
1.1.& 1.2. tone thresholds
- within one session
- over time

1.3 & 1.4. speech thresholds
- within one session
- over time

1.5 & 1.6. tinnitus identification (tinnitometry)
- within one session
- over time

Ad 2.2. Are different approaches of a same physiological phenomenon consistent ?

1.7. tone / speech audiometry
1.8. recruitment assessment
1.9. conventional thresholds / von Békésy thresholds
1.10. prosthetic tone thresholds
1.11. prosthetic speech intelligibility curves
1.12. masking tests

Ad 2.3. Are subjective data concordant with objective data ?

1.13. clinical examination
1.14. impedance measurements / stapedius reflexes
1.15. oto-acoustic emissions: SOAE (spontaneous otoacoustic emissions) - TEOAE (transient evoked oto-acoustic emissions)
1.16. otoacoustic emissions: DPOAE (distortion products otoacoustic emissions)
1.17 BERA (brainstem evoked response audiometry)
1.18 CERA (cortical evoked response audiometry)

Ad 2.4. Are the anamnestic data compatible with the (psycho-)physiological data ?

1.19. tinnitus mentioned already in medical documents prior to context of claim for compensation
1.20. tinnitus mentioned at medical exam for occupational health and safety
1.21. tinnitus mentioned from the 1st contact with the insurance organism
1.22. evidence for therapeutic seek / therapy trial(s)

Ad 2.5. Does the hearing loss show the characteristics of NIHL at functional hearing assessment ?

1.23. type of hearing loss
1.24. severity
1.25. symmetry
1.26. recruitment

Ad 2.6. Has the patient actually been exposed to dangerous occupational noise ?

1.27. type of exposure
1.28. duration of exposure
1.29. SPL levels
1.30. individual technical protection

Ad 2.7. Is the anamnesis and is the history of complaints suggestive for progressive occupational hearing loss ?

1.31. type of hearing complaints
1.32. time history of complaints
1.33. use of protection devices
1.34. use of hearing aids (at work ?, in private life ?)
1.35. use of masking devices for tinnitus

Ad 2.8. Does the functional assessment of tinnitus (tinnitometry) suggest the etiology of cochlear noise damage ?

1.36. pitch matching
1.37. masking possibility and minimal masking level
1.38. loudness matching
1.39. specific characteristics: pulsatile, bitonal…

Ad 2.9. Does the medical history demonstrate compatibility of tinnitus with the etiology of cochlear noise damage ?

1.40. middle ear pathology / surgery
1.41. trauma capitis
1.42. acute acoustic trauma
1.43. inner ear pathology, dizziness, vertigo, fluctuating hearing loss, Ménière, sudden deafness
1.44. eighth nerve pathology, schwannoma
1.45. pharmacology
1.46. poisoning , intoxication
1.47. vascular pathology, hypertension
1.48. neurologic pathology, polyneuropathy, central nervous system disease
1.49. psychiatric pathology

Ad 2.10. Is the anamnesis and is the history of complaints suggestive for tinnitus related to progressive occupational hearing loss ?

1.50. history of tinnitus (onset)
1.51. relation to working activities, private life activities…
1.52. relief conditions

Ad 2.11. Are there convincing objective elements for the nature and severity of impairment / disability / handicap ?

1.53. presence / absence of proven therapeutic seek / demand (medical advice of one / several medical specialties… ; non-medical treatments)
1.54. trial of pharmacological treatment(s)

1.55. personal purchase of physical devices (as e.g. tinnitus maskers)
1.56. consultation of a neuro-psychiatrist
1.57. psychiatric treatment
1.58. psychiatric hospital admission

Ad 2.12. Are there convincing subjective elements for the nature and severity of impairment / disability / handicap ?

1.59. changes in daily life (ceasing specific activities, hobbies)
1.60. sleeping troubles, use of hypnotic drugs
1.61. avoiding specific eliciting or aggravating circumstances
1.62. behavioral changes: irritableness
1.63. neurovegetative symtoms, headache
1.64. influence on mood
1.65. depression, tendency to suicide
(all these to be confronted with objective elements)

3. Interrater reliability

In order to check for agreement between different experts of first level decisions, as well as for concordance in higher level decisions, ten exemplative files were selected within the patient material of the Institute of Occupational Disorders. All were examined by four different medical specialists (oto-rhino-laryngologists) all interested in legal and forensic medicine. They had to make their decision according to the pathway proposed in the protocol. A variant of Cohen's Kappa (Fleiss, 1981) was applied, as this statistical test takes in account the possible agreement between raters by chance (there are no more than 3 choices). It fits the Kappa to the situation of more than two raters. The test reveals a Kappa value of 0,74, demonstrating a high inter-rater consistency at the first level. In all ten cases, the decisions at levels 3 and 4 were identical.

4. Implementation in medicolegal practice

The material consists of 113 consecutive patients with a history of occupational exposure to noise and claiming for compensation for tinnitus and NIHL within the framework of the Belgian insurance system for occupational diseases (Dejonckere & al., 2009). All requests were introduced in the period 2004 - 2009.

In each individual case, a detailed technical inquiry on working conditions and environment was performed by an engineer of the Federal Institute of Occupational Diseases. All patients were also requested to provide a copy of all medical documents in their possession, and - when available - medical files were collected from the Occupational Health and Safety Service (including annual audiometric data).

All patients had an exhaustive otological and audiological investigation within the ENT-department of the Federal Institute of Occupational Diseases, including tone and speech audiometry (prosthetic audiometry when relevant), automatic audiometry (von Békésy), impedance audiometry, evoked response audiometry (including frequency-specific cortical responses to stimuli of 1, 2 and 3 KHz), recording of spontaneous and evoked otoacoustic emissions, and tinnitometry. Combined with the information from the medical history and the medical correspondence and documents, the data of the clinical and instrumental investigations were used to check the 65 items of the level 1 of our decision making system.

According to this decision making system, 35 out of the 113 claimants were recognized as having a tinnitus directly related to their NIHL, and specifically compensated for this tinnitus. Normally the compensation for tinnitus is additional to that for NIHL, but in 23 cases, compensation concerned the sole tinnitus, as the severity of the NIHL was insufficient. Acceptance as an occupational disease automatically implies a proposal for withdrawal from the noisy workplace (with possible occupational recycling and compensation), or a technical adaptation.

As controls, 35 files of patients were selected with also a history of occupational exposure to noise, and also claiming for compensation for NIHL in the same period, but without complaints of tinnitus. The control group was matched for the criterion of a similar (on average) hearing loss at 3 and 4 KHz, accounting for a comparable cochlear damage due to noise. The average thresholds on 3 and 4 KHz for the tinnitus group are 54,83 and 61,17 dB, and for the control group 54,57 and 61,30 dB.

5. Results

5.1 Outcomes of the decision making system

Arguments for a negative decision at level 4, implicating a rejection of the tinnitus component of the claim in 78 claimants, were as follows:

At least one out of the four decisions at level 3 needed to be negative, but it frequently occurred that two or even three of these decisions came out unfavorably.

1. **Reliability**: 38 times negative. This negative decision never occurred as the sole one.
2. **Concomitant occupational NIHL**: 25 times negative, and 2 times as sole negative decision.
3. **Relation Tinnitus-NIHL**: 57 times negative, and 5 times as sole negative decision.
4. **Degree of impairment**: 24 times negative, and 2 times as sole negative decision.

Distribution of allowed impairment percentages are given in the histogram of Fig. 2

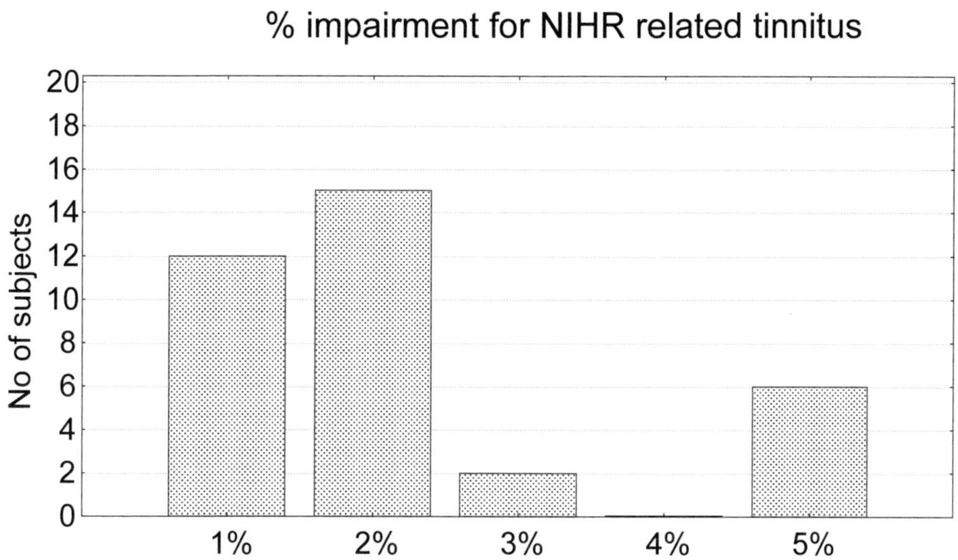

Fig. 2. Distribution of allowed percentages for tinnitus (35 patients). These percentages are in addition to those allowed for hearing loss.

5.2 Characteristics of the tinnitus in the cases considered as related to NIHL and recognized as occupational disease

The tinnitus was bilateral in 31 of the "accepted" cases, and unilateral in 4 cases (3 left, 1 right).

The histogram of Fig. 3 shows the distribution of perceived tinnitus frequency in the 66 investigated ears (tinnitotopy). In most cases tinnitus is located at 4 KHz.

The histogram of Fig. 4 shows the distribution of perceived tinnitus intensities above the pure tone hearing threshold. In average, the tinnitus is perceived 7,20 +/- 3,4 dB above the threshold.

On average, the tinnitus has been lasting for 7,3 years, with a large spreading.

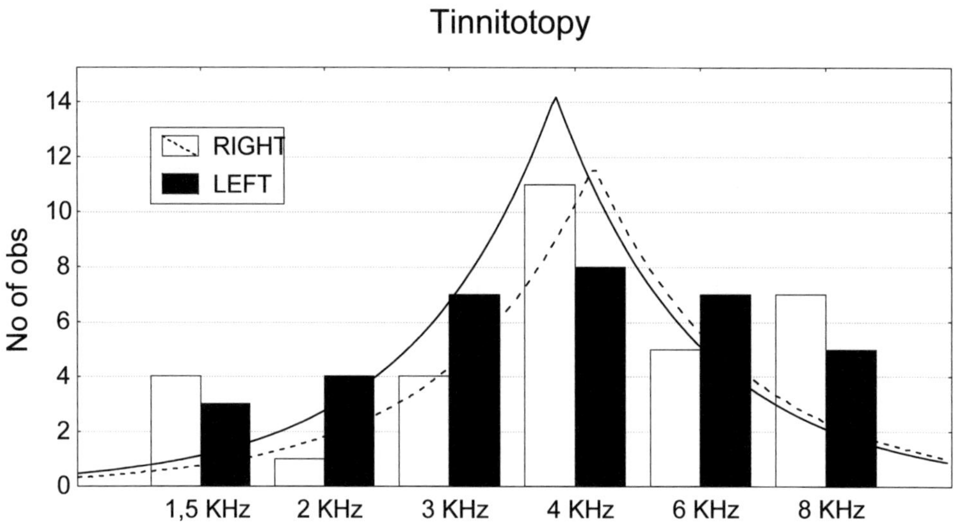

Fig. 3. Distribution of perceived tinnitus frequency in the 66 investigated ears (tinnitotopy) (Lagrange fitting curve).

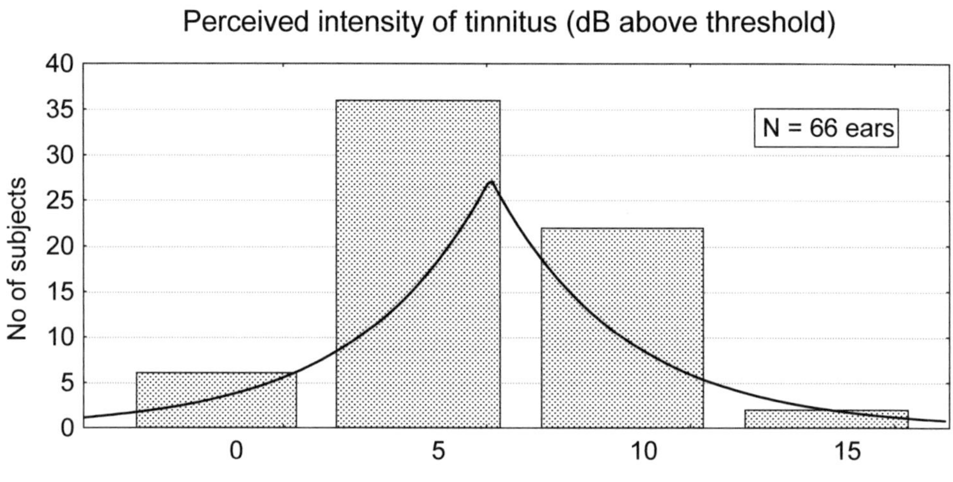

Fig. 4. Distribution of perceived tinnitus intensities above the pure tone hearing threshold (Lagrange fitting curve).

5.3 Comparison with the matched control group

Age

Subjects with NIHL-related tinnitus are slightly younger than control subjects: 48,9 vs. 53,5 years on average (Fig. 5). The difference is significant ($p < ,01$; Mann-Whitney test).

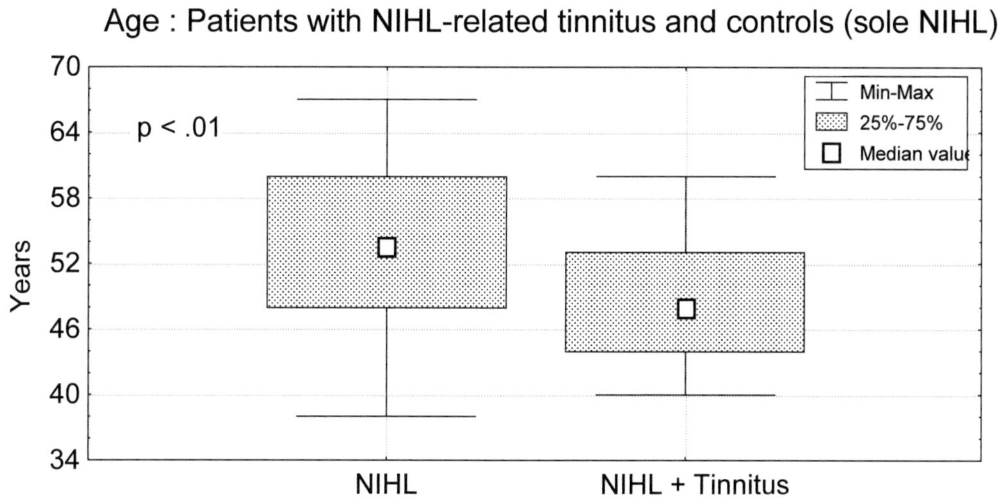

Fig. 5. Age of subjects with NIHL-related tinnitus and control subjects with NIHL but free from tinnitus.

Duration of noise exposure

Duration of noise exposure is slightly less in the tinnitus group than in the control group: 25,7 vs. 28,7 years on average (Fig. 6). However the difference does not reach the ,05 significance level (Mann-Whitney test).

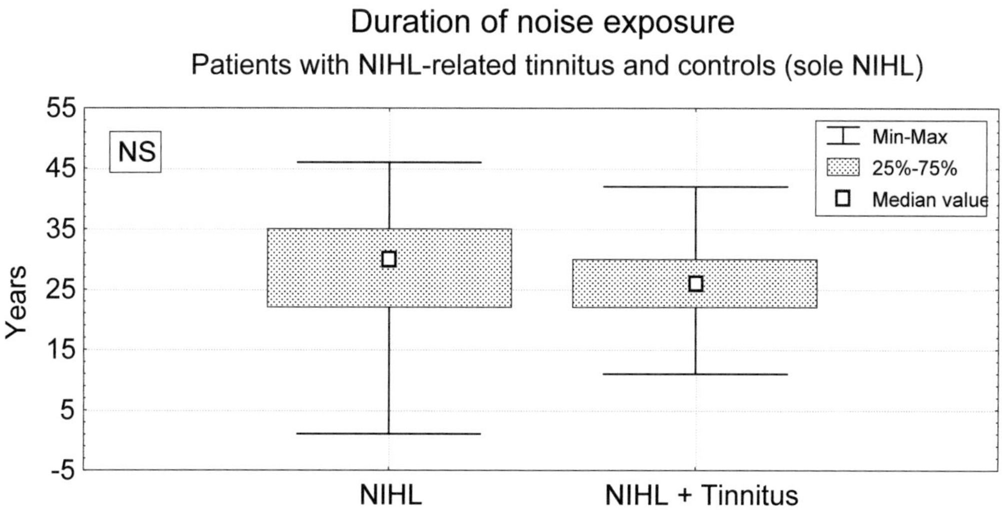

Fig. 6. Duration of noise exposure in the tinnitus group and in the control group.

Pattern of hearing loss

Fig. 7 shows the average hearing levels (+/- 1 S.D.) for 1,2,3,4 and 6 KHz for the subjects with (66 ears) and without (70 ears) tinnitus respectively. Hearing levels on 3 and 4 KHz were used to match the two groups. However, variances differ highly significantly ($p < ,001$) between

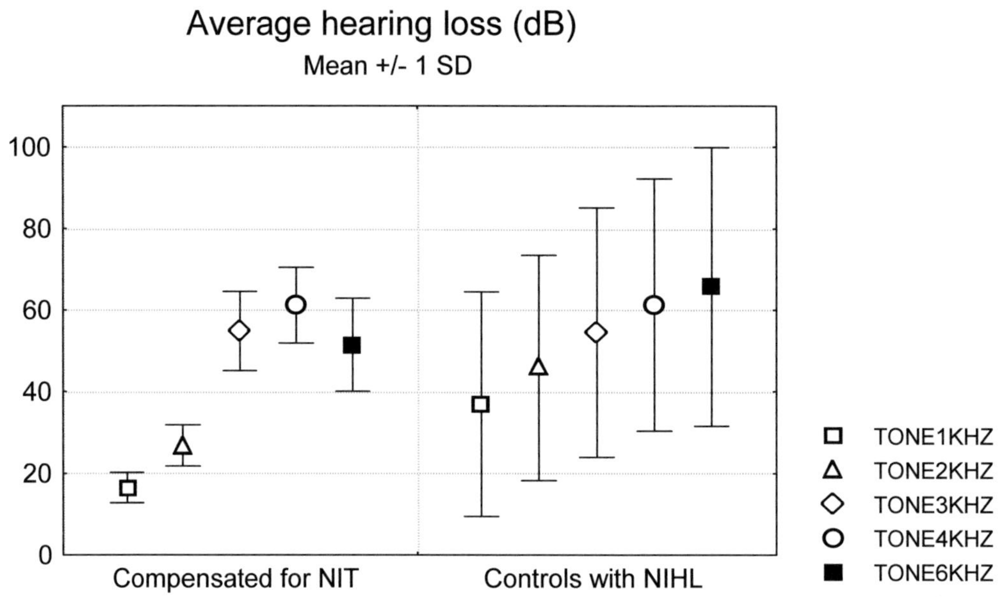

Fig. 7. Average hearing levels (+/- 1 S.D.) for 1,2,3,4 and 6 KHz for the subjects with (66 ears) and without (70 ears) tinnitus respectively. Hearing levels on 3 and 4 KHz were used to match the two groups.

the two groups for all frequencies: spreading is smaller in the tinnitus group. Further a Mann-Whitney test indicates that – except for 3 and 4 KHz - the hearing loss is more pronounced in the group without tinnitus: p is always < ,001. Furthermore, the pattern of the two averaged audiometric curves is different: the typical 4 KHz notch is lacking in the control group. A sign-test reveals that the difference in hearing level between 4 and 6 KHz highly significantly differs between the two groups (p < ,001): in the tinnitus group, the hearing level improves on 6 KHz compared with 4 KHz, while in the control group the 6 KHz value is worse.

DPOAEs

DPOAEs were recorded according to the usual DP-Gram procedure. The distortion product elicited by the non-linear intermodulation between two sinusoids of frequencies f1 and f2 along the basilar membrane was measured at 2f1 – f2 . A fixed ratio of f2/f1 = 1,22 is set for all the measurements and the level of the two pure tones is 70 dB HL. The equipment is able to test frequencies from 1000 to 8000 Hz. According to Attias & al. [7], DPOAEs are considered to be present only if values (in dB SPL) are larger than at least 2 SD above the upper noise floor at the corresponding frequency. A notch (3-4 KHz) in the DPOAEs was observed in 39 out of the 66 ears with tinnitus, but only in 6 out of the 70 control ears (p < ,001: Chi-square test).

6. Discussion

Reliability of the subject

Medico-legal decision making needs to rely upon maximal objectivity. A few basic points are helpful in assisting medical criticism and experience:

1. Reproducibility requires an internal reference. Inconsistent responses are suspicious.
2. When, within an exhaustive assessment, those topics for which the patient's assertion can be objectively controlled systematically demonstrate reliability, it may reasonably be assumed that those for which such an objective control is impossible, are also credible. This is particularly true when the patient ignores which of the items can be objectively controlled.
3. Reports or indications about existence of tinnitus prior to any compensation claim (e.g. in the file of the occupational medicine physician) support reliability.
4. Similarly, documents proving seek for relief of tinnitus before any claim for compensation are highly relevant in this context (repeated medical consulting, acupuncture, purchase of tinnitus maskers, etc.)
5. Verifiable changes in the daily life or behavior of a tinnitus patient may comfort plausibility (e.g. terminating an activity within a choir) and reflect severity as experienced by the patient.

Concomitant occupational NIHL

25 claims were rejected because of lack of concomitant occupational NIHL. A detail to be mentioned is that in order to be considered meaningful, the hearing threshold shift (air conduction) on 4 KHz in the best ear needs to be at least 25 dB above normal value (Ref.: ISO-norm 7029 2nd ed. 2000-05-01). Attias & al. (2001) define NIHL as a hearing threshold more than 25 dB HL at the high frequency range.

Relation Tinnitus-NIHL

Reasons to consider the relation tinnitus-NIHL as improbable referred to medical history and anamnestic data (e.g. onset of tinnitus), clinical and audiological findings, subjective characteristics of tinnitus (e.g. pulsating), tinnitometry (e.g. 125 Hz) together with data obviously pointing to another etiology than NIHL: e.g. sudden deafness, Menière's disease, otosclerosis, trauma capitis, commotio labyrinthi, blast, middle ear disease, hypertension, cerebral MRI-(vascular)lesion, side-effect of drugs.

Degree of severity and allowed impairment/disability %

For reasons of maximal objectivity in determining an impairment percentage, the estimation of the degree of severity needs - particularly in a medicolegal context - to rely as far as possible on factual and verifiable data. Such data are e.g. provided by the extent and intensity of the medical/paramedical help seeking specifically related to the tinnitus, particularly before the claim for compensation was introduced. Also purchase of devices for relieving tinnitus and personal expenses for alternative treatments may be relevant information.

The following rating scale is indicative (all items specifically concern the tinnitus):

Level 0: neither medical nor alternative seeking for help.

Level 1: consulting the home physician, looking for alternative medicine. Treatment with sedatives, hypnotics.

Level 2: consulting an ENT-specialist or a neurologist. Treatment with Betahistine and vasoactive drugs…; physical treatments; tinnitus maskers; psychological treatments…

Level 3: referral to a psychiatrist. Treatment with antidepressive and psychotropic drugs, psychotherapy.

Level 4: psychiatric hospitalization for major behavioral troubles. Treatment with major psychiatric drugs.

In our series, there was only one level 4-case, but – according to the patient himself and to his home physician – the tinnitus was a secondary problem. Three patients were referred to a psychiatrist, but required no more than a short treatment. In the case of a serious psychiatric problem, the medical expertise of a psychiatrist would obviously be requested.
The reason of a negative decision 4 in level 3 ("Is the tinnitus disabilitating, and if so, to what extent ?") was mostly that, when patients were examined, the tinnitus had disappeared or was disappearing. In other cases, patients reported about the tinnitus (besides the hearing loss), but did not consider it as actually disabilitating.

Perceived frequency of tinnitus (tinnitotopy)

Our observation – the correspondence in frequency between audiometric notch and tinnitus – is in agreement with the literature: Okumura & al. (2006) also noticed a strong correlation between tinnitus frequency and hearing loss. The presence of whistling tinnitus was found significantly correlated with high frequency hearing loss (Nicolas-Puel & al., 2006).

Perceived intensity of tinnitus

The observed tinnitus sensation levels are also in agreement with values reported in the literature: those obtained by Andersson (2003) were not higher than 16 dB supraliminal.

Pattern of hearing loss

Our tinnitus and control groups were matched for similar average thresholds at 3 and 4 KHz. This may be interpreted as a similar cochlear damage specifically due to noise, which fits with a comparable duration of noise exposure. Average ages are slightly different (48,9 and 53,5). In normal subjects, this age difference would account for a shift of up to 5 or 6 dB on 6 KHz (ISO-norm 7029 2nd ed. 2000-05-01) but it has been shown that in subjects with NIHL, the superimposed effect of presbycusis in the notch zone (3-4-6 Hz) is considerably reduced (Gates & al., 2000): hair cells lost from one cause cannot be 're-lost again' from another cause. Nevertheless, it seems that the tinnitus group was exposed at a younger age than the control group.
The main audiometric differences between our two groups are:

i. a significantly higher hearing loss at the non-matched frequencies in the control group;
ii. a steeper slope of the curve between 2 and 3 KHz in the tinnitus group (0,028 dB/Hz vs. 0,009 dB/Hz);
iii. a lack of notch effect in the control group.

These findings seem to point out that there is a relationship between the occurrence of tinnitus and a marked imbalance between hearing levels at the different frequencies, particularly 2 and 3 KHz. König & al. (2006) compared 30 patients having noise-induced hearing loss without tinnitus and 41 (non-matched) patients having noise-induced hearing loss with tinnitus. They found that tinnitus patients had less overall hearing loss than patients without tinnitus. Moreover, the maximum steepness of the audiogram was higher in patients with tinnitus (-52,9 +/-1,9 dB/octave) compared to patients without tinnitus (-43,1 +/-2,4 dB/octave).
This abrupt discontinuity in the activity along the tonotopic axis of the auditory system could be a factor facilitating perceptual auditory misinterpretation (tinnitus), as there appears to be a correspondence between audiometric notch and tinnitus frequency.
Differences in the audiometric patterns of the two groups are partially to be explained by concomitance of other hearing pathologies in the control group (nosocusis). A scotopic hearing loss on 3-4 KHz is known to be highly specific of NIHL.

DPOAEs

Hitherto, there have been only a few reports on tinnitus, NIHL and DPOAEs, and they are to some extent controversial (Ozimek & Wicher, 2006). DPOAEs were found to correlate moderately and negatively with the audiometric thresholds (Attias & al. 1998), but Shupak & al. (2007) conclude that, in subjects with beginning NIHL, the DP-gram is not significantly correlated with pure tone audiometry . Attias & al. (2001) as well as Ozimek & Wicher (2006) found in subjects with NIHL and tinnitus a notch shape of the DPOAEs reflecting quite well the hearing loss notch. Our data of the tinnitus group support these last observations. The difference with the control group is probably due to the more severe hearing damage on 1, 2 and 6 KHz .

7. Conclusion

Tinnitus is frequently associated with occupational hearing loss, and can be an additional item of claim in countries applying a specific insurance system for occupational disorders.
As it is not objectivable, tinnitus remains a difficult item for medicolegal assessment and compensation within an insurance context. A decision making system based upon an exhaustive investigation and a 4-level decision structure, proves to be helpful. An aggregate of multiple choice decisions (yes / no / partially) on elementary questions leads to a decision of the next level, which in turn determines – together with the other decisions of the same level - the conclusion at a still higher level. The 4 main decisions at level 3 each pertain to a specific independent aspect, and appear to be in comparable proportions the limiting factor for acceptance of the tinnitus as an occupational disease. A variant of Cohen's Kappa for multiple raters demonstrates high inter-rater consistency at the first level (ten cases, four raters). In all cases, the decisions at higher levels 3 and 4 appear to be identical.
Furthermore, cases with one single negative decision at level 3 are a minority. The analysis of the files where NIHL-related tinnitus was recognized and compensated as an occupational disease show tinnitus characteristics that are in full agreement with what is known from the clinical and epidemiological literature (thus out of medicolegal context). Comparison with a matched group of patients claiming compensation for NIHL without tinnitus reveals that NIHL-related tinnitus is associated with a more specific audiometric profile of cochlear damage due to noise. This specificity mainly concerns the notch on 4 KHz and the steep slope of the audiometric curve between 2 and 3 KHz. Patients with NIHL - related tinnitus have also been exposed on average at a younger age than patients with sole NIHL.
A major advantage with the use of the decision making system is that the final medico-legal decision relies on standardized criteria and becomes perfectly tranparent in case of litigation.
The final aim is maximal equity in compensation.

8. References

Andersson G: Tinnitus loudness matching in relation to annoyance and grading of severity. Auris Nasus Larynx 30: 129-133, 2003.

Attias J, Bressloff I, Reshef I, Horowitz G, Furman V: Evaluating noise induced hearing loss with distortion product otoacoustic emissions. Br J Audiology 32: 39-46, 1998.

Attias J, Horovitz G, El-Hatib N, Nageris B. Detection of noise-induced hearing loss by Otoacoustic Emissions. Noise & Health 3, 12: 19 - 31, 2001.

Coles R. Medicolegal issues. In R Tyler (ed), Tinnitus Handbook. San Diego: Singular Thomson Learning , 2000: pp. 399 - 417.

Dejonckere PH, Lebacq J: Medicolegal decision making in noise-induced hearing loss - related tinnitus. Int Tinnitus J 11: 92-96, 2005.

Dejonckere PH, Coryn C, Lebacq J: Experience with a Medicolegal decision-making system for occupational hearing loss-related tinnitus. Int Tinnitus J 15: 185-192, 2009.

Fleiss JL: Statistical methods for rates and proportions. 2nd Ed. Wiley New York, 1981.

Gates GA, Schmid P, Kujawa SG, Nam B, D'Agostino R: Longitudinal threshold changes in older men with audiometric notches. Hearing Research 141: 220-228, 2000.

König O, Schaette R, Kempter R, Gross M: Course of hearing loss and occurrence of tinnitus. Hearing Research 221: 59-64, 2006.

Nicolas-Puel C, Akbaraly T, Lloyd R, Berr C, Uziel A, Rebillard G, Puel JL: Characteristics of tinnitus in a population of 555 patients: specificities of tinnitus induced by noise trauma. Int Tinnitus J 12: 64-70, 2006.

Nieschalk M, Stoll W. Die Begutachtung von Tinnitus. In Das neurootologische Gutachten. Wolfgang Stoll (ed.) Thieme Verlag, Stuttgart NewYork, 2002, pp. 94 - 98.

Okumura H, Satoshi S, Sato H, Takahashi S. Location of tinnitus frequency examined from the pure tone audiometric pattern. Pract Oto Rhino Laryngol 99(7): 523-530, 2006.

Ozimek E, Wicher A: Distortion product otoacoustic emission (DPOAE) in tinnitus patients. J Acoust Soc Am 119: 527-538, 2006.

Poole K. A review of the current state of knowledge on tinnitus in relation to noise exposure and hearing loss. Research Report HSE 2010 www.hse.gov.uk.

Shupak A, Tal D, Sharoni Z, Oren M, Ravid A, Pratt H. Otoacoustic emissions in early noise-induced hearing loss. Otology & neurootology 28: 745-752, 2007

Part 6

Tinnitus and Metabolic Syndromes

7

Components of Metabolic Syndrome and Their Relation to Tinnitus

Ludovit Gaspar[1], Michal Makovnik[1],
Matej Bendzala[1], Stella Hlinstakova[1],
Ivan Ocadlik[1] and Eva Gasparova[2]
[1]*Second Department of Internal Medicine, University Hospital Bratislava*
[2]*ENT Outpatients Department, Novapharm Bratislava*
Slovak Republic

1. Introduction

Tinnitus is defined as a non-specific symptom characterized as buzzing, whistling, fizzing, ringing or sensing of wide frequency range and different intensity sounds in one or both ears. Tinnitus is a sensation of sound perceived by an individual in the absence of an external sound source. It affects approximately 15% of the population worldwide. Tinnitus is usually connected with many kinds of hearing disturbances, but it could be also a symptom of different other health problems. Metabolic syndrome and its components as arterial hypertension, diabetes mellitus, obesity and dyslipoproteinaemia with arteriosclerosis are important and frequent causes of tinnitus. Due to the high number of heterogeneous etiologic factors in subjective and objective tinnitus a complex approach in differential diagnosis is crucial. Tinnitus can be a concomitant symptom to many disorders of peripheral statoacoustic apparatus. It is necessary to distinguish whether tinnitus is an acute symptom in onset, e.g. in Menière's disease, acute trauma, inflammation of the inner ear, or it is a part of chronic disease otological in origin. Various cardiovascular diseases can be the cause of newly arisen or persistent tinnitus. Among the most important causes there is a reduced perfusion with ischemic changes. Vascular changes can be localized either extra- or intracranially. Among them are stenosis of arteries, haemangioma and glomus caroticum tumours. Changes in the rheology of blood in anaemia or polycythemia can be the cause of tinnitus, as well. It is important to think also about vasculitis as a cause of tinnitus especially among younger patients. Diagnosis of hypertension requires serious and careful approach. The use of a 24-hour ABPM should be considered and carried out as soon as possible in patients with presence of tinnitus. Despite our results are from the limited number of patients with tinnitus, the diagnostic of arterial hypertension is very important, as several prospective studies have reported that ABPM give better prediction of clinical outcomes compared with conventional clinic or office blood pressure measurements. The inner ear, like the brain, is totally lacking in energy reserves. Its metabolism depends directly on the supply of oxygen and glucose from the blood supply. Alterations in glucose metabolism therefore have great potential for disturbing the workings of the inner ear.

2. Classification of tinnitus

a. Objective tinnitus

Objective tinnitus is usually of rhythmical character and can be registered. It can arise from muscle spasms or alteration to the vessels. Although there is a wide spectrum of these disorders, objective tinnitus is not very common, only about 1-2 % of all tinnitus cases (Møller, 2007).

b. Subjective tinnitus

Subjective tinnitus is defined as the perception of sound on the absence of an internal or external sound source. Subjective tinnitus is perceived only by a patient. Its origin is in acoustic analyser or in the brain. Tinnitus itself is not a disease. It is a symptom going along with other diseases. But in fact it can be a dominant sign of the whole clinical picture especially when it is persistent, it has increasing intensity and negative effect on work ability and psychosomatic status. The etiology of a majority of cases is not known (Feldmann, et al., 1992).

It has to be distinguished from acoustic hallucinations as a part of some psychiatric disorders. The most frequent causes of tinnitus are shown in table 1.

Disorders of acoustic analyzer and central nervous system
Alternation of the structures of the inner ear and acoustic nerve
Menière's disease
Infection of the inner ear and sinuses
Acoustic trauma
Chronic noise exposure
Otosclerosis
Neurinoma of the auditory nerve
Arterial hypertension
Arterial hypotension
Diabetes mellitus
Arteriosclerosis
Aneurysm
Disorders of metabolism
Kidney diseases
Head and neck trauma
Cervical spine and temporomandibular joint diseases
Hematological diseases with the change in viscosity of blood and changes in microcirculation
Exogenous noxious substances - nicotine, alcohol, caffeine
Medications: antibiotics, NSAIDs, antidepressants, cytostatics, furosemide, oral contraceptives
Industrial toxins - heavy metals, carbon monoxide, aniline, benzol
Artificial sweeteners containing aspartame
Lues
Autoimmune diseases

Table 1. The most frequent causes of tinnitus

Tinnitus is described as an unwelcome symptom. Tinnitus can be an attendant phenomenon in specific diseases, but in some cases his origin and cause is unknown. Through the precise etiology in most cases is unknown, an abnormal interaction between peripheral and central auditory pathways is believed to play a role in tinnitus development. Tinnitus is associated with the most important symptoms in neurootology, besides vertigo, nausea and hearing loss. There are many forms of subjective tinnitus witch can occur with different severity.

The parameters of tinnitus that require identification are intensity, location, duration, quality, maskability and rebound. The patient may report the intensity as mild, moderate or severe. Various grading systems have been used to provide a means of communication between the patient and examiner.

The biological mechanisms leading to the perception of tinnitus are still not completely understood. Increasing agreement, however, posits that different forms of tinnitus may differ in their patophysiological mechanisms. Also generally accepted is that most forms of subjective chronic tinnitus are the consequence of central nervous system reorganization processes induced by altered peripheral auditory and somatosensory input. Peripheral deafferentation may result in an imbalance between excitatory and inhibitory function, causing maladaptive plastic changes in the structural and functional organization of the auditory system at several levels (dorsal cochlear nucleus, inferior colliculus, medial geniculate body and auditory cortex).

Sudden sensorineural hearing loss is defined as hearing loss equal to or greater than 30 dB at three or more consecutive frequencies, the onset of which takes place over a period 3 days of fewer. In most cases, it is severe, nonfluctuating, unilateral and idiopathic. Approximately one-third of cases are accompanied by complains of tinnitus, dizziness and ear fullness.

3. Obesity and metabolic syndrome

Obesity is a chronic progressive disease characterized by the accumulation of fat tissue with multiple organ-specific pathological consequences which has a significant impact on morbidity, as well as the quality and length of the obese individuals` life.

The prevalence of obesity in many European Union countries has tripled since the year 1980 and further is increasing alarmingly, only during the last 10 years the number of obese has increased by 10 to 40%. Obesity is responsible for 2-8% of the costs and 10 to 13% of deaths in the region of the European Union. Overweight and obesity in the European region has more than 50% of the population. 20% of children and adolescents are overweight and a third of them are obese (Branca et al., 2007). Data from United States show that 65% of the local population has excess weight and 31% are obese. These data highlight the epidemic situation of obesity, and therefore the WHO considers reversing of this trend as one of its priorities (Haslam & James, 2005).

In Table 2 are examples of the connection of obesity with a number of associated diseases and conditions.

An abdominal adiposity as the cardiovascular risk factor is associated with components of metabolic syndrome, namely with insulin resistance, disturbed glucose metabolism, hypertension and dyslipidemia. With these components it is very closely linked to acceleration of the process of atherosclerosis and its serious systemic complications. It is important that the effect of these components (factors) together in mutual combination is not simply added, but multiplied.

Cardiovascular disease: coronary artery disease, myocardial infarction, systemic arterial hypertension, atherogenic dyslipidemia, stroke
Oncologic diseases: endometrial and ovarian cancer, prostate, breast, rectum, kidney, liver, gallbladder cancer
Diabetes mellitus type 2 and insulin resistance
Hepatic steatosis
Osteoarthropathy
Deep vein thrombosis and pulmonary embolism
Chronic renal failure
Polycystic ovary syndrome
Hyperuricemia
Gallstones
Reproductive disorders
Lumboischialgic syndrome
Ventilation pulmonary complications
Sleep apnea syndrome
Psychological and social problems
Complications in pregnancy
Complications in the perioperative period

Table 2. Obesity is connected with a number of associated diseases and conditions

Obesity and overweight are important markers of coronary heart disease and lead to an increase in cardiovascular and cerebrovascular morbidity and mortality (Narkiewicz, 2006). Adipose tissue is an endocrine organ. It synthesizes and releases several specific components, eg. cortisol, estrogen, leptin, adiponectin, resistin, nonesterified free fatty acids, interleukin 6 (IL-6), tumor necrosis factor alpha (TNF-alpha), plasminogen activator inhibitor-1 (PAI-1) and others. These influence and are in relationship to the overall cardiometabolic risk in an individual patient (Bonora, 2006). Many epidemiological studies show that prevalence of hypertension increases progressively with increasing BMI (body mass index) as for men as well as in women. Relationship between BMI and blood pressure (BP) is stronger for systolic (SBP) as the for diastolic (DBP) blood pressure. Data from the NHANES III study (Foley et al., 2005) clearly indicate, that the risk of hypertension developing is closely relate to the waist, as well as waist / hip ratio (WHR). In general, it is estimated that in about 75% of men with hypertension and in 65% of women with hypertension is present overweight or obesity. Data from the Finnish population studies suggest up to 85% prevalence of hypertension in persons with BMI over 25 kgm^2 (Kastarinen et al., 2000). Obesity and particularly central obesity leads to increased cardiovascular risk. Results of population studies suggest that at least two thirds of the prevalence of hypertension can be directly attributed to the impact of the obesity (Krauss et al., 1998).

3.1 Pathophysiological changes in the cardiovascular system in obesity

In the obesity there is a change in the fundamental characteristics of circulation, as heart stroke volume and cardiac output, peripheral vascular resistance, changes in the flow distribution. It leads, in association with other risk factors, to the development of arterial hypertension and coronary heart disease. The degree of obesity correlates directly with cardiac output and is inversely associated with systemic vascular resistance. The increase in cardiac output in obese is resulting from an increased stroke volume, while heart rate does not correlate with BMI (Kurtz & Klein, 2009; Messerli et al., 1981). Stroke volume is probably associated with an increased intravascular volume (non-obese 50 ml/kg vs. obese 75 ml/kg). Central type of obesity, however, is associates with lower cardiac output and higher total peripheral vascular resistance, and the deviation of above parameters is even increased by the mental stress. Splanchnic blood flow is increased by 20%, flow through the kidneys and the brain remains unchanged (Jern et al., 1992). Distribution of body fat influences the muscle morphology and density of the muscle capillary network. Persons with a higher waist circumference have less type I muscle fibers and more type IIB fibers. Type IIB has about 20 to 30% lower density of capillary network. In the case of stress response can be expected to lower vasodilative response in the muscles, followed by the less efficient splanchnic vasoconstriction in stress defense response. Abdominal obesity has been associated with increased activity of hypothalamic-pituitary-adrenal axis, which is a major part of the neuroendocrine system that controls reactions to stress and defense reaction (Howell et al., 2004; Rahmouni et al., 2005).

There is a higher cardiac output in obese individuals, higher circulating intravascular volume and increased oxygen consumption, but total blood flow in relation to body weight is reduced. An increased sympathetic activity is also common in obesity, which may in long-term activation cause hypertension by the peripheral vasoconstriction and increased tubular reabsorption. Studying regional sympathetic activity in obese subjects was found an excess of noradrenaline in relation to the kidneys as a key organ of cardiovascular homeostasis. Both obesity and hypertension lead to the development of left ventricular hypertrophy and subsequent diastolic dysfunction (Redon et al., 2008).

Adipose tissue is through several mechanisms, directly integrated into the pathogenesis of hypertension. These mechanisms include alteration of renin-angiotensin-aldosterone system (RAAS), increased activity of the sympathetic nervous system, insulin resistance, leptin resistance, alteration of coagulation and inflammatory factors in the development of endothelial dysfunction. Activation of adipose RAAS is involved particularly in the creation and development of hypertension in the central (visceral) type of obesity. Especially in this type of obesity is increased level of plasma aldosterone (Goodfriend & Calhoun, 2004). The cause of the increase in production can be potent mineralocorticoid-releasing factors, or effect of oxidised linolenic acid compounds on aldosterone synthesis (Goodfriend et al., 2004).

Leptin is a link between adiposity and increased sympathetic activity. In addition to effects on appetite and metabolism, leptin increases blood pressure by the sympathetic activation in hypothalamus (Carlyle et al., 2002). Understanding the role of leptin in the pathophysiology of sympathetic overactivity in obese patients facilitates the concept of selective leptin resistance. Leptin-induced increase in renal sympathetic activity and blood pressure is mediated by the ventromedial and dorsolateral hypothalamus (Marsh et al., 2003). Selectivity refers to the different signaling pathways distal to the leptin receptor. Enzyme fosfoinozitol-3 kinase is an important intracellular signaling pathway for the control of renal sympathetic systeme, because inhibition of this enzyme reduces sympathetic activity. Melanocortin system is also an important regulatory axis, with the effects on renal sympathetic and blood pressure (da Silva et al., 2004).

Hypertension contributes to increased cardiovascular and cerebrovascular morbidity and mortality through effects on atherogenesis by multiple mechanisms: it leads to endothelial dysfunction with impairment of responses to vasodilatating substances, to increased vascular permeability for macromolecules (also for lipoproteins), to the increased production of vasoconstrictor endothelin and to increased adherence of leukocytes, also to the remodeling of smooth muscles in large arteries, whereas in small arteries it causes increased vascular tone. An increase in angiotensin II level and PDGF act as growth factors for smooth muscle cells of the media, their effect is potentiated by the endothelin. Phenotypic change of vascular smooth muscle cells may also occur, thus increasing their proliferative potential and their proliferative response to growth factors (Fábryová, 2008).

Endothelial dysfunction in terms of reduced reactivity to nitric oxide (NO) is a typical abnormality in obesity. Impaired endothelium is a major risk factor for cardiovascular diseases because it leads to structural changes such as the rebuilding of the intima and media of wall of blood vessels. Strong factor for the development of endothelial dysfunction is the increased production of endothelin-1 in patients with hypertension and obesity. Blockade of endothelin receptor-A induces significant vasodilation in subjects with overweight and obesity, but not in the case of normal-weight patients with hypertension (Cardillo et al., 2004).

Obesity is associated with several structural and functional changes in kidneys. RAAS and sympathetic activation increases the levels of plasma aldosterone with consequent increases in renal sodium reabsorption, which leads to impaired sodium excretion and the expansion of circulating blood volume. Obesity can also cause structural changes in the kidney, leading to chronic renal failure with a further increase in blood pressure. Mechanic pressure of abdominal adipose tissue in the visceral type of obesity may have also a role in renal impairment. Besides sympathetic autonomic nervous system also the leptin plays a role, which acts directly by increasing oxidative stress with a demonstrable increase in isoprostane levels in blood and urine, increased lipid peroxidation products in kidney tissue and decreased renal activity of aconitase (Beltowski et al., 2004). Obesity can cause glomerular hyperfiltration, abnormal albuminuria and progressive loss of kidney function due to focal segmental glomerulosclerosis (Kambham et al., 2001). Number of nephrons is reduced in patients with primary hypertension (Keller et al., 2003). In patients with pre-existing renal disease, obesity accelerates the progression of the disease and renal insufficiency (Praga et al., 2000). Structural kidney damage may further increase blood pressure and predispose to cardiovascular events.

3.2 Pathophysiological changes in the respiratory system in obesity

Obesity, especially abdominal type, is associated with deterioration of pulmonary function. Abdominal obesity is limiting diaphragm descent and expansion of lung parenchyma, in comparison with total adiposity, which compresses the chest wall. Compression of the lung parenchyma leads to decrease in expiratory reserve volume and functional residual capacity, which reduces the compliance of respiratory system. In obese patients with normocapnia breath work is at rest increased by 30%, in physical activity may be insufficient breath work limit for further increase in minute output with development of the relative hypoventilation. Products associated with abdominal type of obesity, such as serum leptin, CRP, leukocytes, fibrinogen have an inverse relationship to FEVl, therefore, inflammation may be connection between altered respiratory function and mortality (Schünemann et al., 2000; Sin & Man, 2003).

3.3 Obesity and sleep apnea syndrome

Obesity is associated with sleep apnea syndrome and obesity hypoventilation syndrome (Pickwickian syndrome, alveolar hypoventilation). In sleep apnea syndrome, pharyngeal airway passive collapse during deep stages of sleep, causing snoring and intermittent airway obstruction. The resulting hypoxia and hypercapnia cause disturbance of the normal sleep quality and subsequent daytime sleepiness, development of pulmonary and systemic vasoconstriction, polycythemia and right heart failure. Relative hypoventilation may cause progressive desensitization of respiratory centers to hypercapnia, followed by respiratory insufficiency.

Obesity hypoventilation syndrome is one of several diseases associated with chronic hypercapnia and alveolar hypoventilation. Obesity is associated with increased risk of alveolar hypoventilation and carbon dioxide retention. Hypoxemia and increased alveolar-arterial oxygen gradient in patients with obesity hypoventilation syndrome draws attention not only to alveolar hypoventilation, but also the ventilation - perfusion mismatch.

Patients with chronic obstructive pulmonary disease and sleep apnea, as well as patients with obesity hypoventilation syndrome in addition to systemic arterial hypertension also have high prevalence of pulmonary arterial hypertension (Nowbar et al., 2004; Šimková, 2009).

It is clear that hypertension dependent on obesity is a multifactorial disease. Obese individuals tend to hypertension, but vice-versa, hypertensive individuals tend to weight gain. As the Framingham and Tecumseh studies also showed, that future weight gain is significantly greater in hypertensive than in normotensive persons. This finding indicates that the hypertensive patients, even with normal weight are at increased risk of developing obesity and other complications resulting from it (Julius et al., 2000).

The link between increased BMI and mortality is documented by the analysis of 57 prospective studies (Flegal et al., 2007). For both sexes, the lowest mortality was found in BMI from 22.5 to 25 kg/m^2. In all age categories 35 to 59 years, 60 to 69 year, 70 to 79 y. and 80 to 89 years was revealed significant increase in mortality in persons with BMI 25 to 50 kg/m^2. BMI in its entirety from 15 to 50 kg/m^2 was associated almost linearly with systolic and diastolic blood pressure. Obesity was significantly associated with diabetes. This explains the positive and approximately log-linear relationship of BMI and an increase in the number of deaths due to ischemic heart disease with a 40% increase in CHD mortality for an increase in BMI for every 5 kg/m^2. The same results were found for stroke. Mortality due to heart failure and hypertension was also strongly associated with higher BMI.

Different groups of antihypertensive agents differ significantly in their metabolic effects. It is important to consider significant differences in this effect between different types of pharmaceuticals within the group itself, which is particularly true for beta-blockers. From the centrally acting antihypertensive drugs, it has been proven beneficial effect for weight reduction in moxonidine. Administration of ACE inhibitors and AT1 blockers is significantly reducing the risk of type 2 diabetes. Their complex beneficial effects affect not only the hypertension itself, but also the whole cascade of metabolic changes; therefore preparations that affect the renin-angiotensin system are essential treatment of hypertension in obesity and metabolic syndrome. From the group of sartans, telmisartan is unique substance in this respect, which significantly improves insulin sensitivity. From the drugs which may adversely affect weight and cause its sharp increase are particularly significant psychiatric medications. This undesirable side effect can be observed mainly in the traditional neuroleptics and tricyclic antidepressants (Svačina, 2002).

4. Metabolical disease

Extensive laboratory tests should be performed at the time of the general medical evaluation in addition to sugar and thyroid metabolism to evaluate the status of serum cholesterol and triglycerides level. Triglyceride levels have been reported to be considered in evaluating patients with inner ear or Menière's disease. There has been evidence of a positive experience in a small but significant number of patients, more male than female, for the identification of these factors in association with secondary endolymphatic hydrops. Significantly, the incidence of subjective idiopathic tinnitus in patients with diabetes mellitus has been infrequent in the series. The subjective idiopathic tinnitus was cochlear and was influenced positively by glucose control.

Nutritional deficiencies and imbalances are considered of significance in relation to ear disease and specifically for complaints of sensorineural hearing loss, vertigo and tinnitus. The clinical history is correlated with laboratory test results, which attempt to identify imbalances, deficiencies, and/or excesses of nutrients that are considered to upset the biochemical balances of the hearing organ resulting in malfunction of hearing and/or balance process. Impaired carbohydrate metabolism and its control have been identified in a significant number of patients with Menière's disease. The identification by clinical history and laboratory tests including determination of insulin levels, followed up by specific treatment to correct such an imbalance, is reported to significantly improve symptoms of endolymphatic hydrops (sensorineural hearing loss, vertigo, tinnitus). Hyperinsulinemia has three different effects: sodium retention within cochlear duct with a resulting endolymphatic hydrops, vasoconstriction caused by the effect of prolonged hyperinsulinemia in long term hypertrophy of arterial smooth muscles cells, and cholesterol formation and atherosclerosis within the arterial walls of the branches internal auditory artery. Impairment of glucose metabolism is of particular significance in the aged population. The chemical attachment of the sugar glucose to proteins without the aid of enzymes may contribute to age-related impairment of both cells and tissues. In this nonenzymatic process, glucose is described to have the capability of attaching itself to several sites along any available peptide chain. This process is called nonenzymatic glycosylation of certain proteins in the body. Glucose may play a role in tissue changes associated with normal aging. Elevated cholesterol and triglycerides levels have been reported with fluctuant hearing loss, vertigo, and tinnitus. A triad of elevated levels of insulin and triglycerides and impaired glucose tolerance has been reported, particularly in obese patients. The identification of these abnormalities combined with dietary control has been reported to result in considerable control of fluctuant sensorineural hearing loss, vertigo, and tinnitus. Association of a triad of hypertension and atherogenic diet and chronic noise exposure acts synergistically for the development of a sensorineural hearing loss (Pillsbury, 1986).

5. Arterial hypertension and tinnitus

Stabilization of the symptoms of hypertension has been found to have a significant positive influence on treatment in general and for the following clinical types of subjective idiopathic tinnitus (cochlear tinnitus, vestibular tinnitus and central tinnitus). Tinnitus has been found to be a "soft" sign of cerebro-vascular disease and secondary endolymphatic hydrops. For these clinical types of tinnitus as well as tinnitus of specific causes, blood pressure control has afforded appreciable control. Ear and/or head blockage complaints should also be respected as an accompaniment of a possible "symptom less" hypertension. The term essential hypertension has been applied to idiopathic hypertension. Essential hypertension is marked by its heterogeneity and multifactorial nature. There have been identified clinical similarities between essential hypertension and subjective idiopathic tinnitus. Classically, patients have reported problems of tinnitus in association with elevated blood pressure. These are usually anecdotal reports, in the past, control of hypertension resulted in significant control of subjective idiopathic tinnitus. Therefore, the concept of and role of hypertension in the production and control of tinnitus is and old one. What is new is to reverse the thinking of hypertension as resulting in tinnitus to that of the presence of tinnitus as reflecting possible hypertension. In a significant number of tinnitus patient, the early identification of tinnitus has been accompanied by an elevation in blood pressure. Blood pressure control not only has resulted in a reduction in tinnitus intensity, but also has provided hearing conservation as well as the alteration or control of progression of complaints of cerebrovascular disease, cardiovascular complications, e.g. myocardial infarction, congestive heart failure, vertigo, progressive sensorineural hearing loss, and ear and/or head blockage. In a significant number of tinnitus patients, any or all of these symptoms together with that of tinnitus have been found to present as a symptoms complex reflecting an early manifestation of hypertension.

The essential quality of the hypertension requires investigation and attention by the internist. This is a particularly evident among aged patients. In a significant number of patients in the aged group have either an acute onset of tinnitus and/or exacerbation of chronically present tinnitus accompanied by an elevation of blood pressure. The clinical correlation of hypertension and the tinnitus onset has also been found in the younger population, i.e., below age 40, but less frequently. Epidemiological studies concerning the relationship of blood pressure elevation with age concluded that this relationship has, as yet, not been determined (Morris, 2007). In some patients, blood pressure does increase with middle age. Some studies (Miall et al., 1967), did show positive correlation with advancing years. Tinnitus may be an early symptom that has wide-reaching consequences in a significant number of the aged population. The heterogeneity and multifactorial elements involved in essential hypertension, particularly in the aged, can explain the great degree of variability of its in tinnitus patients with or without hypertension. What is significant is that tinnitus may be a very early sign of onset of hypertension and/or an inadequate blood pressure control.

Sodium and water retention and a reduction in urinary excretion are of particular significance for those subjective tinnitus patients who may have a vestibular asymmetry with or without subjective complaints of vertigo and who are diagnosed with secondary endolymphatic hydrops. Secondary endolymphatic hydrops may be considered in the subjective tinnitus patient to be a mechanism for gradual progressive sensorineural hearing loss. Its control has, in a significant number of patients, resulted in satisfactory tinnitus control. Significant is that the initial blood pressure increase, which has been shown to originate in an area other than that of the kidney, is, however, maintained by the kidney by complex changes occurring in renal dynamics, as manifested by fall in renal blood flow and renin and increase in total renal vascular resistance.

Psychobiologic factors are significant for both subjective idiopathic tinnitus and essential hypertension. Essential hypertension can serve as can no other disease as model of the multifactorial nature of all diseases in which complex interactions between inherited, environmental, social, cultural, experiential, physiological and biochemical factors occur. No single cause of essential hypertension appears to exist, no qualitative, discontinuous alteration has been discovered to explain its etiology or pathogenesis. Like essential hypertension, subjective tinnitus demonstrates heterogeneity of its manifestations, both for the mechanism involved in its production and/or its clinical manifestation. Both conditions share common factors including socio-economic, cultural, ethnic, behavioural and psychological factors.

Consideration should be given to the group of tinnitus patients for whom adequate sleep is accompanied by reduction in tinnitus. It has been known for some time, that behavioural states can affect blood pressure levels, which are much lower in sleep, than in the waking state. In both states, psychological factors are significant. In essential hypertension, the psychological factors alone are not considered sufficient to explain the predisposition to or pathogenesis of the disorder. The physiologic heterogeneity that results in hypertension is reflected in the psychological heterogeneity. Future clinical investigations of the relationship between the sensory and affect components in both these health problems may clarify diagnosis, treatment and control of subjective idiopathic tinnitus. In both conditions, social and psychological factors interfere in the clinical results of the prescribed treatment. Hypertensive patients often do not follow treatment and medication regiments. Similarly, tinnitus patients may not accept a treatment method that may provide tinnitus relief, because the recommendations may not fulfils the patient's expectation for cure or provide sufficient control.

When developing treatment and control methods for both tinnitus and essential hypertension, the physician must consider that both are disorders not only of adaptation but also of regulation, which may be reflected in one or more systems. This has already been established for hypertension, and it may apply to tinnitus.

6. Ambulatory Blood Pressure Monitoring (ABPM) in patients with tinnitus

The aim of our study was to assess the prevalence of unknown arterial hypertension in patients with tinnitus.

Patients and methods: We investigated 18 patients (8 female, 10 male) with median age 46 (age spread 34 - 64 years) with tinnitus lasting from 4 months to 6 years. Known history of arterial hypertension and antihypertensive medication was an excluding criterion. After otorhinolaryngologic examination and estimating the tinnitus magnitude and frequency with pure tone audiometry with Interacoustics, Denmark AC40 audiometer (figure 1), we performed ambulatory blood pressure monitoring (ABPM) using CardioSoft - TONOPORT V - General Electric, USA device with oscilometric BP measuring (figure 2).

The general medical-physical and otorhinolaryngologic examination should always precede the neurootologic investigation. The physical examination includes attention to the identification of any deformity or limitation of movement of the head, neck, spinal column, and joints. Inspection of the scalp and skull are supplemented by careful palpation to attempt to identify a localized thickening of the skull, abnormal scalp vessels, depressions of the skull, abnormal contours and asymmetry of the skull, past craniotomy, and/or other operative scars. In the presence of a large head, particularly in an adult, percussion is performed for evidence of possible hydrocephalus. Auscultation with a stethoscope is performed over the skull and neck for bruits. The effect on the bruit of head turning and compression of the carotid artery, right and left, back and forwards is noted.

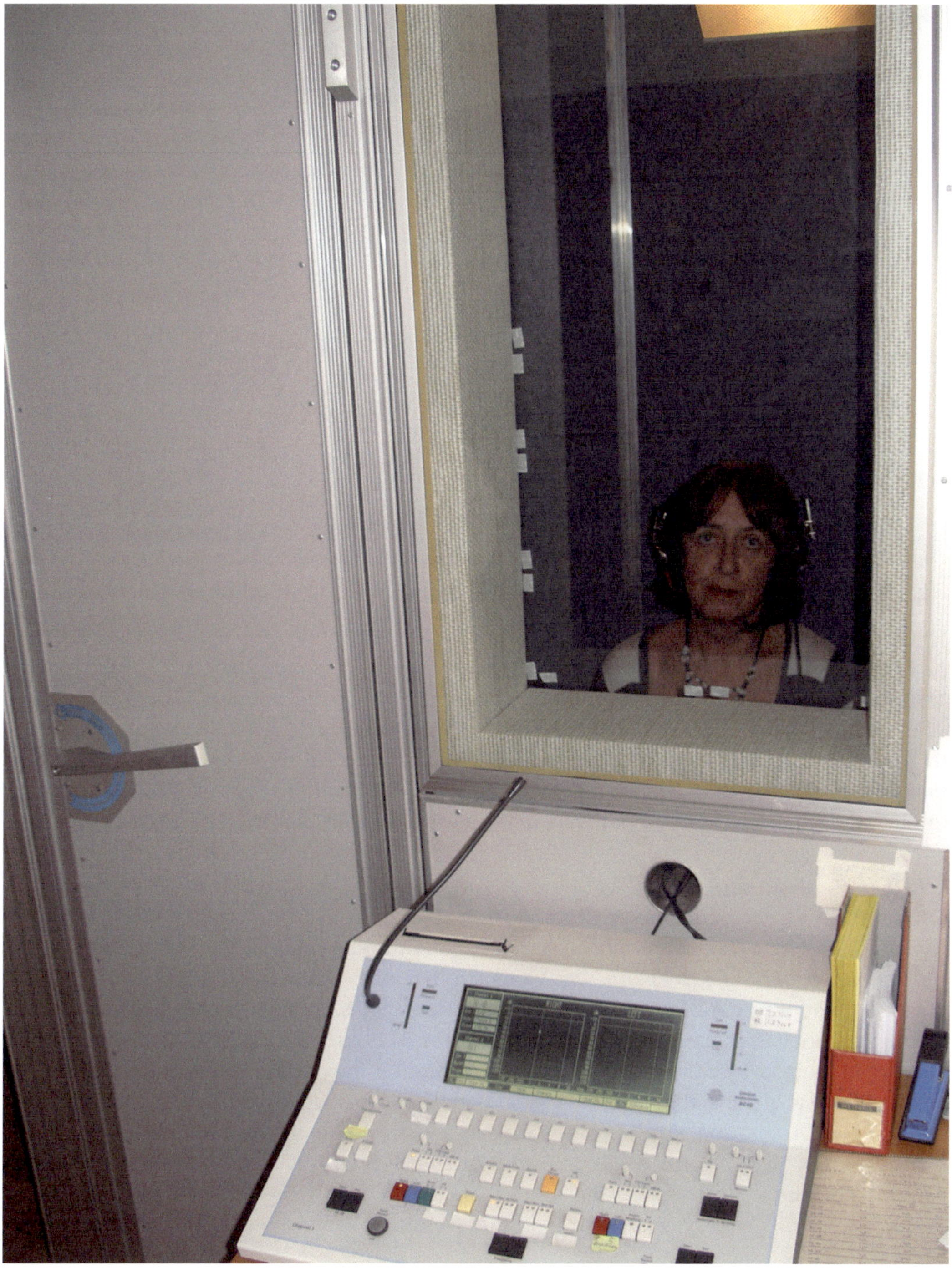

Fig. 1. Clinical Audiometer AC 40, Interacustics, Denmark used for measurement of thresholds of audibility and specification of tinnitus.

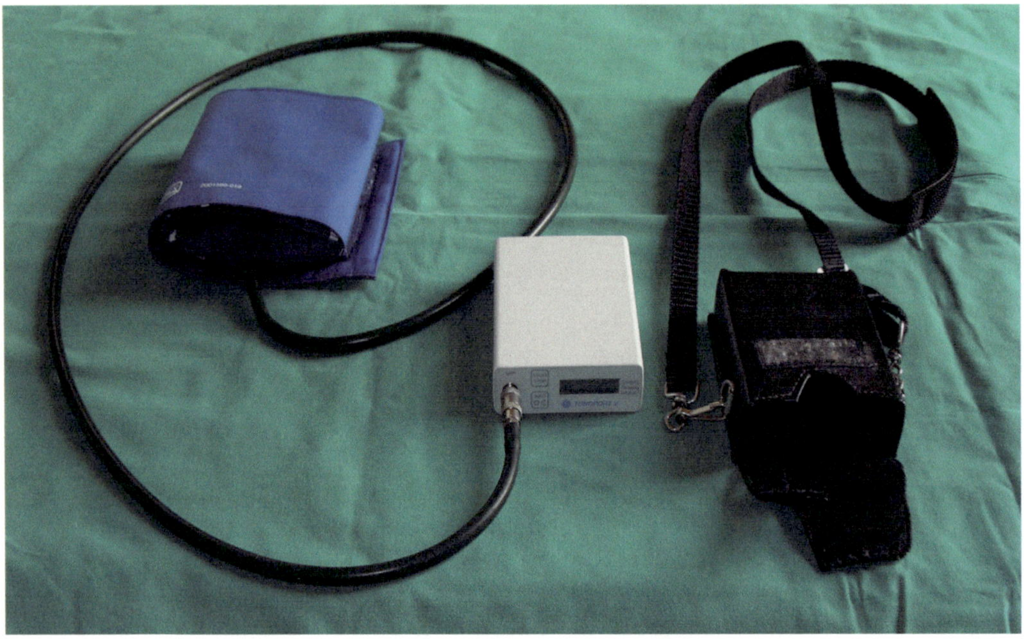

Fig. 2. Cardiosoft - Tonoport - V - General Electric, USA device used for 24-hours ABPM

Figure 3 shows audiogram with bilateral symmetric perceptive acoustic disorder. Then we performed internal examination and indicated a 24-hour ambulatory blood pressure monitoring (ABPM). We used for this examination Cardiosoft-Tonoport V-General Electric, USA device, which uses oscillometric method of measurement of blood pressure. None of the group member has previous known diagnosis of arterial hypertension, or use of any medication altering blood pressure level. As some medications can evoke or strengthen tinnitus thoroughly, history of patient's medication is very important (Holcát, 2007).

6.1 Results of our study

The average values of blood pressure during a 24-hour ABPM were 140/89 mmHg. In daytime phase and nighttime phase the average values were 143/91 mmHg and 130/81 mmHg, respectively. Diurnal sign was vanished in 5 individuals (28%). 6 persons (33%) had normotension during a 24-hour ABPM. 12 persons (66%) had hypertension with an average blood pressure values more than 130/80 mmHg for 24-hours. All records had a good quality what permits interpretation of ABPM profile including mean daytime, nighttimes, 24-hour measurement and diurnal pattern loss. Based on these results, we followed the patients from the group with abnormal ABPM results further and also with repeat measurement of casual blood pressure; we confirmed the arterial hypertension with necessity of antihypertensive drug treatment.

7. Discussion

Due to the high number of heterogeneous etiologic factors in subjective and objective tinnitus a complex approach in differential diagnosis is crucial. Tinnitus can be a concomitant

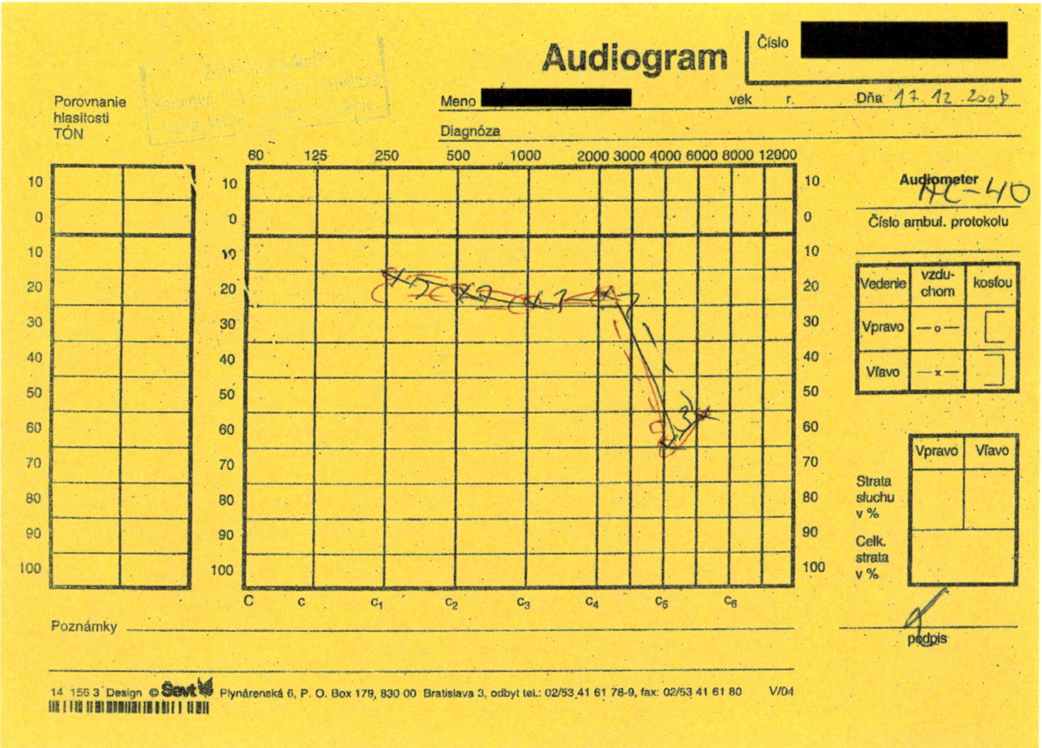

Fig. 3. Audiogram with bilateral symmetric perceptive acoustic disorder, decrease of hearing thresholds bilateral (red line - right ear, blue line - left ear) in frequency 3000-6000 Hz

symptom to many disorders of peripheral statoacoustic apparatus. It is necessary to distinguish whether tinnitus is an acute symptom in onset, e.g. in Menière's disease, acute trauma, inflammation of the inner ear, or it is a part of chronic disease otological in origin (Møller, 2003). Various cardiovascular diseases can be the cause of newly arisen or persistent tinnitus. Among the most important causes there is a reduced perfusion with ischemic changes. Vascular changes can be localized either extra- or intracranially. Among them are stenosis of arteries, haemangioma and glomus caroticum tumours. Changes in the rheology of blood in anaemia or polycythemia can be the cause of tinnitus, as well. It is important to think also about vasculitis as a cause of tinnitus especially among younger patients (König et al., 2006).

The process of differential diagnosis usually starts at the otolaryngologist but interdisciplinary approach to the patient is needed.

Tinnitus is frequent among patients with arterial hypertension, diabetes mellitus, thyroid gland disorders, rheumatologic and neurologic diseases. Two-thirds of our 18 patients with tinnitus had newly diagnosed hypertension during a 24-hour ABPM.

The mean duration of tinnitus in our group was 4 years (range 4 months to 6 years). As none of the patients had formerly diagnosed hypertension, it is likely that hypertension arose after the onset and duration of tinnitus. Diagnosis of hypertension requires serious and careful approach and the use of a 24-hour ABPM should be considered and carried out as soon as possible in patients with presence of tinnitus. Despite that our results are from the limited number of patients with tinnitus, the diagnostic of arterial hypertension is very important, as several prospective studies have reported that ABPM give better prediction of clinical outcomes compared with conventional clinic or office blood pressure measurements (Staessen et al., 1999).

Tinnitus is a stressor, which can significantly decrease the quality of life, and it can cause serious mental disorders. Some circumstances (stress, acute infection, anaemia) can lead to increase of duration and intensity of tinnitus. Concomitant sleep disorders, anxiety, despair, frustration and depression as well as aggressiveness are related to higher frequency of psychosomatic disorders (Crönlein et al., 2007). Tinnitus then becomes a complex health problem and symptom becomes syndrome (Langguth et al., 2007). Due to the increased incidence of arterial hypertension in this group of patients a 24-hour ABPM is fully indicated. Approximately 17% of the population of USA and Europe and 15% of the population worldwide had manifestation of some form of tinnitus. Only half of them sought for medical help. In 15 - 20% of cases, tinnitus affects quality of life, with repercussions involving sleep habits, concentration, emotional stability and social activities (Axelsson & Ringdahl, 1989; Dobie, 1999). The degree of discomfort caused by this symptom may be mild when perceived by an individual only in particular situations (occurring among approximately 7% of the individuals); moderate when the individual is aware of its existence but does not feel bothered by it; intense when the unpleasant sensation is disturbing and has a negative effect on activities of daily living. It is severe when the symptom becomes unbearable, ever-present and ceaselessly affecting the activities of daily living with concomitant psychic problems. The degree of discomfort, intolerance, or incapacity caused to the individual is often not related to the loudness (sensation of intensity) of the tinnitus (Prestes & Gil, 2009).

8. Conclusions

1. Our result suggests that undetected hypertension is very often in patients with tinnitus.
2. Arterial hypertension is one of many factors involved in tinnitus origin and continuing.
3. ABPM is a suitable tool for hypertension detection and management also in this group of patients.
4. Diagnosing and treating arterial hypertension may not influence tinnitus presence and intensity, but can avoid serious complications of hypertension e.g. stroke, myocardial infarction, heart or renal failure.
5. Diabetes mellitus as one of the components of metabolic syndrome with its complications as micro- and macroangiopathy, cardiovascular autonomic neuropathy is an important and frequent etiologic factor of tinnitus.

9. References

Axelsson, A. & Ringdahl, A. (1989). Tinnitus--a study of its prevalence and characteristics. *British Journal of Audiology,* Vol.23, No.1, (February 1989), pp. 53-62, ISSN 0300-5364

Beltowski, J.; Wójcicka, G.; Marciniak, A. & Jamroz, A. (2004). Oxidative stress, nitric oxide production, and renal sodium handling in leptin-induced hypertension. *Life Sciences,* Vol.74, No.24, (April 2004), pp. 2987-3000, ISSN 0024-3205

Bonora, E. (2006). The metabolic syndrome and cardiovascular disease. *Annals of Medicine,* Vol.38, No.1, (2006), pp. 64-80, ISSN 0785-3890

Branca, F.; Nikogosian, H. & Lobstein, T. (2007) The Challenge of Obesity in the WHO European Region and the Strategies for Response, In: *World Healt Organisation 2007,* 12.09.2010, Available from http://www.euro.who.int/document/E90711.pdf

Cardillo, C.; Campia, U.; Iantorno, M. & Panza, J. (2004). Enhanced vascular activity of endogenous endothelin-1 in obese hypertensive patients. *Hypertension,* Vol.43, No.1, (January 2004), pp. 36-40, ISSN 1524-4563

Carlyle, M.; Jones, O.; Kuo, J. & Hall, J. (2002). Chronic cardiovascular and renal actions of leptin: role of adrenergic activity. *Hypertension,* Vol.39, No.2, (February 2002), pp. 496-501, ISSN 1524-4563

Crönlein, T.; Langguth, B.; Geisler, P.; & Hajak, G. (2007). Tinnitus and insomnia *Progress in Brain Research,* Vol.166, (2007), pp. 227-233, ISSN 0079-6123

da Silva, A.; Kuo, J. & Hall, J. (2004). Role of hypothalamic melanocortin 3/4-receptors in mediating chronic cardiovascular, renal, and metabolic actions of leptin. *Hypertension,* Vol.43, No.6, (June 2004), pp. 1312-1317, ISSN 1524-4563

Dobie, R. (1999). Indirect A review of randomized clinical trials in tinnitus. *The Laryngoscope,* Vol.109, No.8, (August 1999), pp. 1202-1211, ISSN 0023-852X

Fábryová, Ľ. (2008). Vzťah viscerálnej obezity ku kardiometabolickým faktorom. *Via practica,* Vol.5, No.3, (2008), pp. 122-125, ISSN 1336-4790

Feldmann, H.; Lenarz, T. & von Wedel, H. (1992). *Tinnitus,* Georg Thieme Verlag, ISBN 313-770-0027, Stuttgart, Germany

Flegal, K.; Graubard, B.; Williamson, D. & Gail, M. (2007). Cause-specific excess deaths associated with underweight, overweight, and obesity. *JAMA: The Journal of the American Medical Association,* Vol.298, No.17, (November 2007), pp. 2028-2037, ISSN 1538-3598

Foley, R.; Wang, C. & Collins A. (2005). Cardiovascular risk factor profile and kidney function stage in the general population. *Mayo Clinic Proceedings,* Vol.80, No.10, (October 2005), pp. 1270-1277, ISSN 0025-6196

Goodfriend, T. & Calhoun, D. (2004). Resistant hypertension, obesity, sleep apnea, and aldosterone: theory and therapy. *Hypertension,* Vol.43, No.3, (March 2004), pp. 518-524, ISSN 1524-4563

Goodfriend, T.; Ball, D.; Egan, B.; Campbell, W. & Nithipatikom, K. (2004). Epoxy-keto derivative of linoleic acid stimulates aldosterone secretion. *Hypertension,* Vol.43, No.2, (February 2004), pp. 358-363, ISSN 1524-4563

Haslam, D. & James, W. (2005). Obesity. *Lancet,* Vol.366, No.9492, (October 2005), pp. 1197-1209, ISSN 0140-6736

Holcát, M. (2007). Tinnitus and diabetes. *Vnitřní Lékařství,* Vol.53, No.5, (May 2007), pp. 534-536, ISSN 0042-773X

Howell, S.; Sear, J. & Foëx, P. (2004). Hypertension, hypertensive heart disease and perioperative cardiac risk. *British Journal of Anaesthesia,* Vol.92, No.4, (April 2004), pp. 570-583, ISSN 0007-0912

Jern, S.; Bergbrant, A.; Björntorp, P. & Hansson, L. (1992). Relation of central hemodynamics to obesity and body fat distribution. *Hypertension,* Vol.19, No.6, (June 1992), pp. 520-527, ISSN 0194-911X

Julius, S.; Valentini, M. & Palatini, P. (2000). Overweight and hypertension : a 2-way street?. *Hypertension,* Vol.35, No.3, (March 2000), pp. 807-813, ISSN 1524-4563

Kambham, N.; Markowitz, G; Valeri, A.; Lin, J. & D'Agati, V. (2001). Obesity-related glomerulopathy: an emerging epidemic. *Kidney International,* Vol.59, No.4, (April 2001), pp. 1498-1509, ISSN 0085-2538

Kastarinen, M.; Nissinen, A.; Vartiainen, E.; Jousilahti, P.; Korhonen, H.; Puska, P. & Tuomilehto. (2000). Blood pressure levels and obesity trends in hypertensive and normotensive Finnish population from 1982 to 1997. *Journal of Hypertension,* Vol.18, No.3, (March 2000), pp. 255-262, ISSN 0263-6352

Keller, G.; Zimmer, G.; Mall, G.; Ritz, E. & Amann, K. (2003). Nephron number in patients with primary hypertension. *The New England Journal of Medicine,* Vol.348, No.2, (January 2003), pp. 101-108, ISSN 1533-4406

König, O.; Schaette, R.; Kempter, R. & Gross, M. (2006). Course of hearing loss and occurrence of tinnitus. *Hearing Research,* Vol.221, No.1-2, (November 2006), pp. 59-64, ISSN 0378-5955

Krauss, R.; Winston, M. & Fletcher, B. (1998). Obesity : impact on cardiovascular disease. *Circulation,* Vol.98, No.14, (October 1998), pp. 1472-1476, ISSN 1524-4539

Kurtz, T. & Klein, U. (2009). Next generation multifunctional angiotensin receptor blockers. *Hypertension Research: Official Journal of the Japanese Society of Hypertension,* Vol.32, No.10, (October 2009), pp. 826-834, ISSN 1348-4214

Langguth, B.; Kleinjung, T.; Fischer, B.; Hajak, G.; Eichhammer, P. & Sand, P. (2007). Tinnitus severity, depression, and the big five personality traits. *Progress in Brain Research,* Vol.166, (2007), pp. 221-225, ISSN 0079-6123

Marsh, J.; Fontes, M.; Killinger, S.; Pawlak, D.; Polson, J. & Dampney, R. (2003). Cardiovascular responses evoked by leptin acting on neurons in the ventromedial and dorsomedial hypothalamus. *Hypertension,* Vol.42, No.4, (October 2003), pp. 488-493, ISSN 1524-4563

Messerli, F.; Christie, B.; DeCarvalho, J.; Aristimuno, G.; Suarez, D.; Dreslinski, G. & Frohlich, E. (1981). Obesity and essential hypertension. Hemodynamics, intravascular volume, sodium excretion, and plasma renin activity. *Archives of Internal Medicine,* Vol.141, No.1, (January 1981), pp. 81-85, ISSN 0003-9926

Miall, W.; Heneage, P.; Khosla, T.; Lovell, H. & Moore, F. (1967). Factors influencing the degree of resemblance in arterial pressure of close relatives. *Clinical Science,* Vol.33, No.2, (1967), pp. 271-283, ISSN 0143-5221

Møller, A. (2003). Pathophysiology of tinnitus. *Otolaryngologic Clinics of North America,* Vol.36, No.2, (April 2003), pp. 249-266, ISSN 0030-6665

Møller, A. (2007). Tinnitus: presence and future. *Progress in Brain Research,* Vol.166, (2007), pp. 3-16, ISSN 0079-6123

Morris, J. (2007). Uses of Epidemiology. *International Journal of Epidemiology,* Vol. 36, No.6, (2007), pp. 1165-1172, ISSN: 0300-5771, 1464-3685

Narkiewicz, K. (2006). Obesity and hypertension - the issue is more complex than we thought. *Nephrology Dialysis Transplantation,* Vol.21, No.4, (February 2009), pp. 264-267, ISSN 0931-0509

Nowbar, S.; Burkart, K.; Gonzales, R.; Fedorowicz, A.; Gozansky, W.; Gaudio, J.; Taylor, M.& Zwillich, C. (2004). Obesity-associated hypoventilation in hospitalized patients: prevalence, effects, and outcome. *The American Journal of Medicine,* Vol.116, No.1, (January 2004), pp. 1-7, ISSN 0002-9343

Pillsbury, H. (1986). Hypertension, hyperlipoproteinemia, chronic noise exposure: is there synergism in cochlear pathology?. *The Laryngoscope,* Vol.96, No.10, (October 1986), pp. 1112-1138, ISSN 0023-852X

Praga, M.; Hernández, E.; Herrero, J.; Morales, E.; Revilla, Y.; Díaz-González, R. & Rodicio, J. (2000). Influence of obesity on the appearance of proteinuria and renal insufficiency after unilateral nephrectomy. *International Kidney International,* Vol.58, No.5, (November 2000), pp. 2111-2118, ISSN 0085-2538

Prestes, R. & Gil, D. (2009). Impact of Tinnitus on Quality of Life, Loudness and Pitch Match, and High-Frequency Audiometry. *International Tinnitus Journal,* Vol. 15, No.2, (2009), pp. 134-138, ISSN 0946-5448

Rahmouni, K.; Correia, M.; Haynes, W. & Mark, A. (2005). Obesity-associated hypertension: new insights into mechanisms. *Hypertension,* Vol.45, No.1, (January 2005), pp. 9-14, ISSN 1524-4563

Redon, J.; Cifkova, R.; Laurent, S.; Nilsson, P.; Narkiewicz, K.; Erdine, S. & Mancia, G. (2008). The metabolic syndrome in hypertension: European society of hypertension position statement. *Journal of Hypertension,* Vol.26, No.10, (October 2008), pp. 1891-1900, ISSN 0263-6352

Schünemann, H.; Dorn J.; Grant, B.; Winkelstein, W. & Trevisan, M. (2000). Pulmonary function is a long-term predictor of mortality in the general population: 29-year follow-up of the Buffalo Health Study. *Chest,* Vol.118, No.3, (September 2000), pp. 656-664, ISSN 0012-3692

Šimková, I. (2009). *Pľúcna hypertenzia očami kardiológa,* SAP - Slovak Academic Press s.r.o., ISBN: 978-80-8095-051-4, Bratislava, Slovakia

Sin, D. & Man, S. (2003). Impaired lung function and serum leptin in men and women with normal body weight: a population based study. *Thorax,* Vol.58, No.8, (August 2003), pp. 695-698, ISSN 0040-6376

Staessen, J.; Thijs, L.; Fagard, R.; O'Brien, E.; Clement, D.; de Leeuw, P.; Mancia, G.; Nachev, C.; Palatini, P.; Parati, G.; Tuomilehto, J. & Webster, J. (1999). Predicting cardiovascular risk using conventional vs ambulatory blood pressure in older patients with systolic hypertension. Systolic Hypertension in Europe Trial Investigators. *JAMA: The Journal of the American Medical Association,* Vol.286, No.6, (August 1999), pp. 539-546, ISSN 0098-7484

Svačina, Š. (2002). *Obezita a psychofarmaka,* Triton, ISBN: 80-7254-253-2, Prague, Czech Republic

Part 7

New Alternative Treatments of Tinnitus

8

Home Medical Device for Tinnitus Treatment

Martin Lenhardt
Biomedical Engineering, Otolaryngology, Emergency Medicine,
Virginia Commonwealth University, Richmond VA,
USA

1. Introduction

1.1 A tinnitus definition

Tinnitus is almost exclusively defined as ringing in the ear(s); more common in the popular than the professional literature since the turn of the century. It is now well recognized that tinnitus is chiefly neural, that is a perception being in one or both ears. This is not to deny cochlear tinnitus or the role of the cochlea in the tinnitus process. It is also typical to define tinnitus as a phantom sound with no external stimulus; also suggesting tinnitus arises in the central nervous system. The phantom descriptor is somewhat problematic (Shulman, 1995); however external sound can and does influence the perception of tinnitus and is a common therapeutic treatment in the form of masking. Further, that means the perception of tinnitus is interactive with external ambient sound. If sound levels are dramatically reduced as in echo free space (anechoic) normal hearing young individuals will generally report tinnitus like perceptions without sensations. The first in a series of studies Heller and Bergmann, (1952) reported almost 94% of normal hearing subjects experienced hearing sounds in a sound attenuated chamber (ambient level of 15-18 dB SPL) after just a few minutes. This finding was repeated but to a lesser degree in three studies (Del Bo et al., 2008; Knobel and Sanchez, 2008; Tucker et al., 2005) in which a 64-68 % of the subjects reported tinnitus. Most interestingly, if attention was redirected away from the auditory modality, the percent responding was less than half (45%). If the subjects were engaged in a cognitive task the percent report tinnitus was <20%. It is not surprising that attention or top down processing plays a role in tinnitus with normal hearing individuals since it is a major factor in segregating those who are bothered or not by their tinnitus (Erlandsson et al., 1992). For those that are not bothered by their tinnitus, the typical response is I do not pay attention to it.

There are no published reports of tinnitus being induced in the almost absolute silence, in human terms, in anechoic space. The room in the Del Bo et al., (2008) study is termed a sound proof chamber and also an anechoic chamber; it may have been anechoic with sound attenuation below minimal audible fields. Anechoic space is valuable component in an assessment of silence induced tinnitus since the sound levels are generally less than the air reference of 0.0002 dynes/cm^2. While antidotal in nature, I have a vivid memory of my first experience in an anechoic chamber as a graduate student at Florida State University. I walked out on a wire mesh since there were Fiberglas sound wedges below as above and around me. Once the doors were shut I immediately heard my physiological noise of respiration etc. I spoke and it appeared to me that my words were sucked away from my mouth, then, I heard a high frequency hissing seemingly in the middle of my head which I now identify as tinnitus. Upon exiting the chamber all such perceptions ceased. Re-entering the hissing returned as did my sense of bodily noises. The three other graduate students in the lab had the same experience as did other visiting students. We thought this was a common experience not worthy of a formal report. My hearing was at 0 dB HL up to 8 kHz (highest measured) and my minimal audible angle at 2 kHz was < 4^0. A few years later my high frequency hearing was measured and it too was normal up to 20 kHz. I had no more than a cursory understanding of tinnitus and concluded at the time the critical factor in its appearance was the lowered ambient noise of the chamber. With this experience in mind, I must conclude that tinnitus is naturally induced by silence. I have never experience the same tinnitus perception is single or double walled acoustic enclosures with less attenuation.

Absolute silence can also be achieved with eight nerve section. Tinnitus is generally not eliminated, but can be increased by this procedure (Cope et al, 2011) although the effect was found to vary from increased to decreased tinnitus or no effect (Mollar et al., 1993). Tinnitus can be associated with severe deafness and can generally be ameliorated to degree with the electrical stimulation of a cochlear implant (Amoodi et al., 2011; Arndt et al., 2011; Pan et al., 2009).

What then is the mechanism that produces tinnitus with just being in silence or immediately having an eight nerve sectioning, this cannot be the result of complex neural plastic changes in the brain, it is most likely a release from neural inhibition in the peripheral neural structures, probably acting the spiral ganglia by the central auditory system. This would account for the rapid turn on/off when stepping out of anechoic space and back in.

In addition there may be an unmasking of non-lemniscal pathways, again under the influence of the central nervous system. Moller et al., (1992) reported tinnitus patients summed somatosensory stimulation (mild shock to the medial nerve) with an auditory tone which resulted in increased loudness perception. This multimodal effect is seen in young children but not adults. The non-lemniscal pathway is multimodal and the likely candidate for this effect in tinnitus patients. That pathway has a subcortical input into the limbic system and direct input into the auditory association cortex. Whether the non-lemniscal pathway can be activated by just silence has not been studied. This pathway is involved in orientation and would certainly respond to abrupt silence.

Could this pathway be switch on and off with just stepping in and out of anechoic space? Perhaps this is but one element in a cascade of effects inducing the perception of tinnitus. The artificial nature of anechoic space must activate the limbic system and in particular the amygdala. Input to the amygdala is both subcortical (non-lemniscal pathways) and cortical via the classical auditory pathways. These pathways are termed the low and high road respectively by LeDoux (1990). The amygdala is active in severe disabling tinnitus and plays a notable role in contributing to tinnitus annoyance first postulated by Shulman and Goldstein (1996).

Tinnitus is thus a perception without a sensation, that is nonetheless interactive with external sound conditions, generated by the brain.` It is the brain component (both auditory and non-auditory) that appears to be implicated much more so than the ear in the perception of tinnitus in normal hearing individuals and likely those suffering long term hearing loss. It should be apparent, then, that treatment strategies must involve neural mechanisms to be effective and masking meets that criterion in that it has central neural effects (Goldstein et al., 2001).

1.2 Neuroscience of treatment

Tinnitus can be present in individuals with normal hearing; however normal hearing measurement does not always indicate fully intact hair cells (Bredgerg, 1967) or a spinal ganglia free of deaffrination or even cochlea free of dead regions (Weisz et al., 2006). High frequency audiometery on tinnitus patients revealed 12 of 18 had threshold elevation in the high frequency region (10, 12, 14, 16 kHz) in one study (Shim et al., 2009). Goldstein et al., (2006) reported high hearing loss common in severe disabling tinnitus. Thus tinnitus can exist in individuals even if hearing appears unremarkable in the conventional audiometric range and some hearing loss in the very high frequencies may be more commonly present than previously believed (Goldstein et al., 2005). Further, there may be neuroplastic changes in the brain regions that code these very high frequencies, which may contribute to the tinnitus percept. Very high frequency hearing loss (>10 kHz) might benefit from very high frequency sound therapy (Goldstein et al., 2006) including ultrasonic masking Meikle et al., 1999; Lenhardt, 2003).

Overwhelmingly, hearing loss is often associated with tinnitus and it appears to be the key factor triggering the events that lead to tinnitus in humans and animals. The most frequent cause of hearing loss is intense noise which is often characterized as a high frequency loss of hearing behaviorally and a loss of hair cells and changes in the nerve and auditory synapses in the brain. Spontaneous firing rates tend to increase in the first auditory brain synapse (dorsal and ventral cochlear nucleus) as well as in the midbrain (inferior colliculus) and auditory cortex (primary and secondary)[Wienbruch et al., 2006; Eggermont and Roberts 2004]. Tinnitus neural induced changes are not limited to the classical pathways but also present in the non-classical or non-lemnsical pathways (Mollar et al., 1992) Both pathway have input into the limbic system (LeDoux, 1990) and it is the involvement of this system that form the final common pathway in tinnitus (Shulman 1995; Shulman and Goldstein 2006; Shulman et al., 2009).

The change in neurons' spontaneous firing rates along the neuraxis is also accompanied by changes in the neural tuning properties of neurons representing the peripheral region of the hearing loss (Schaetta and Kempter, 2009). The neuromechanisms that give rise to neuro hyperactivity have not been identified but some form of increased gain in the central nervous system is likely, which suggests that additional stimulation covering the effect frequency region might form the basis of sound therapy.

Norena and Eggermont (2005) reported that cats exposed to a traumatizing noise and immediately placed in a 40 dB high frequency sound environment had much less hearing loss compared with similarly exposed cats placed in a quiet environment. The hearing loss in the quiet reared cats ranged from 6 to 32 kHz with the loss, on average, 40 dB. In contrast, the hearing loss in the high frequency environment cats was restricted to 6-8 kHz at a level near 35 dB. Despite the restricted hearing loss for the high frequency stimulated cats in the 6-8 kHz range, no auditory cortical reprogramming was found, suggesting that the high frequency stimulation prevented the expected reorganization. It would seem then an effective treatment for tinnitus in humans would be very high frequency stimulation at a moderate level covering the tinnitus pitch match and the tinnitus spectrum (Schaette et al., 2010)

Encouraged by the Norena and Eggermont's (2005) study high frequency stimulation was applied with tinnitus patients and matched controls with similar sensorineural hearing loss and no history of tinnitus (Goldstein et al., 2005. The results revealed that high frequency stimulation for 5-8 weeks dramatically reduced the level of sound needed to mask tinnitus and thresholds of hearing improved by 5-25 dB suggesting plastic changes had occurred in the central nervous system. The animal study (Norena and Eggermont; 2005) demonstrated that sound therapy can prevent brain reprogramming as a result of one intense noise exposure; thus preserving hearing that would likely have been lost. The human data with people having long term hearing loss and some with severe tinnitus, suggest that the brain can reprogram back, modifying the neural state again, and as a result, making masking more effective at lower levels and improving hearing. Hearing improvement due solely to listening to high frequencies via the UltraQuiet system could generate skepticism; nonetheless, the limited data is very suggestive of threshold improvement due to reverse neuroplasticity in the high frequencies which did not exceed 25 dB. Further the concept is consistent with conventional auditory theory; however sampling variability is clearly a concern, resolvable with an expanded data base.

Only a few decades ago most neural scientists believed that the adult brain was hard wired, now it is well accepted the adult brain is plastic and capable of reprogramming after sensory or motor loss or with learning (Syka et al., 2003). Neural maps change with experience. Hearing loss triggers a reprogramming in the auditory cortex which results in a change in frequency response. With noise induced hearing loss, cortical neurons sensitive to the loss reprogram lower in frequency. Somehow the high frequency stimulation therapy maintains or re-establishes the original neural map. Reduced inhibition is likely the active factor in the cortical affecting the periphery to achieve enhanced hearing.

High frequency sound therapy can restore or even improve hearing by preventing auditory cortical reorganization, that is to say, the auditory cortex contributes to sound sensitivity at the ear. If the auditory cortex is ablated, the audiogram is about 25 dB poorer (see Heffner and Heffner, 1986; 1995 for reviews). The assumption is that the cortex, or its actions (efferent control), exerts an influence on hearing level at the neural periphery. Changes in hearing threshold indirectly implied central changes have taken place as a result of therapy.

2. Medical masking devices for tinnitus

There exist a number of devices for the treatment of tinnitus, however the US Food and Drug Administration (FDA) identified only two, hearing aids and maskers. Combination devices are a merge of a hearing aid and a masker.

2.1 Limitations

Hearing aids are designed to amplify speech sounds and are generally limited in high frequency (<10 kHz) fidelity. Hearing aid use has been reported to be of benefit in adjusting to tinnitus particularly when combined with counseling, since tinnitus evokes a variety of emotional reactions and quality of life issues. Thus a device designed to maximize speech perception as a result of hearing loss is used to treat tinnitus. Increasing the stimulation to the brain appears to be the principal mechanism that induces suppression and or accommodation to tinnitus. Relief from the effects of tinnitus is possible for some, but long term use of hearing aids does not appear to be efficacious for most tinnitus patients. The lack of high frequency energy in hearing aids may limit their success as maskers (Schaette et al., 2010). Combination devices may have more utility (Sweetow and Sabes, 2010) and flexibility in fitting individuals with tinnitus. The use of music in a wearable combination device may be relaxing, but unless the upper frequency limit covers the tinnitus spectrum, the effectiveness may be reduced unless the music is customized (Starackle et al., 2010; Wilson et al., 2010).

Maskers are wearable devices that produce a sound band to mask the tinnitus and through use, produce some measure of tinnitus inhibition. Wearable maskers have been available for the last forty years (Vernon and Meikle, 2000; 2003) and produce about 70% complete masking. Only 10% achieve no masking while the remainder exhibit diminished tinnitus perception. Maskers only cover the tinnitus and do not treat the cause. Maskers can aid in tinnitus habituation but generally they are used at a low volume for that purpose. In the table below, the experience at the Tinnitus Clinic at the Oregon Health and Science University (Vernon and Meikle, 2003) reveals that most patients can get partial or complete masking. The masking efficiency of a commercial high frequency product, UltraQuiet, has comparable efficiency and is an end element in the new technology presented herein (see Table I). Masking alone is not sufficient; the sound must also interact with the brain to reduce the effects of tinnitus.

masking by wearable devices

	Vernon Meikle survey	UltraQuiet
• complete masking	70.5	75
• partial masking	19.6	15
• no masking	9.9	10

Table 1. The wearable masking devices (maskers, hearing aids and combination devices) yielded some degree of masking to 90% of the tinnitus patients in the Oregon survey. UltraQuiet, the end component in the new home based tinnitus system present here had the same level of effectiveness in masking. Long term compliance is a problem for all such devices.

2.2 Economics

Hearing aids and custom maskers are expensive which can limit their utilization in the tinnitus population. Even when purchased, if these devices may be less successful over time, and if so, the patient will possibly become discouraged and abandon the approach that once was successful. It is most important for devices to be part of a structure tinnitus therapy program. Tinnitus devices are also expensive to design, achieve regulatory approval, manufacture, distribute and support.

2.3 Patient preferences

Since tinnitus has no known cure, a variety of treatments from pharmaceuticals to psychotherapy have be suggested; some health care providers still only offer the advice to live with it, thus tinnitus patients in the age of worldwide interaction through the web, are often weary of new treatment approaches, especially expensive ones. Effective tinnitus approaches require patience, perseverance, commitment and discipline. Nonetheless, the typical patient is looking for a cure not a long term treatment. The tinnitus device should be considered only a tool not a solution in and of itself. The tool must be used regularly for full benefit (Del Bo and Ambrosetti 2007).

2.4 Innovation based on best practices and science

Treatment of tinnitus with high frequency signals that cover the tinnitus pitch frequencies (areas of hearing loss) and higher has been shown to be effective using behavioral and imaging studies(Goldstein et al., 2001;2005;Shulman et al., 2004). Nonetheless, the compliance of patients has been less than expected (~75% improvement) outside the research laboratory environment. There is a need for a home based unit that will provide the needed time of treatment to insure success. It is hypothesized that a stand-alone home unit will lead to a greater success rate in treating tinnitus, especially in environments lacking audiological infrastructure and /or professional supervision. Tinnitus devices, dissimilar to hearing aids, are more strictly regulated. The UltraQuiet device is the interface to the patient in a new home unit to be described and that interface has received regulatory clearance.

2.5 UltraQuiet

UltraQuiet is a tinnitus therapy product that provides patterned auditory stimulation in the high audio and into ultrasonic ranges (10-22 kHz) using a bone conduction transducer; and is based on the work of Lenhardt (2003), demonstrating ultrasonic perception by humans. UltraQuiet therapy differs from conventional maskers by providing very high frequency (5-22 kHz) sound therapy. In UltraQuiet therapy, the auditory stimulation is processed music that has been pre-filtered and up shifted in pitch using amplitude modulation (upper sideband). Music was selected as the core of the stimulus since it was found to be more effective tinnitus masker than noise (see Wilson et al., 2010 for review) since music engages more central and cognitive processes. The tinnitus treatment stimulus was produced using Kyma Version 5 software with a Capybara 320 Sound Computation Engine (Symbolic Sound Corporation, Champaign, IL) and stored on a compact disk (CD). The CD signal was fed into a custom-made amplifier delivered to the skin off the head in the mastoid region using a piezoelectric bone conduction transducer. The transducer was held in place by a plastic headband found to have comparable force as a standard metal audiometric bone conduction headband. Although the stimulus is presented on only one side of the head, it is heard binaurally through bone conduction, although it is about 5 dB sensation level (SL) more intense on the fitted side. In UltraQuiet therapy, the processed and frequency shifted music is presented at 12 dB SL for minimum periods of 1 hour twice weekly with daily use encouraged. The goal is to effect changes in the central nervous system mechanisms of tinnitus, resulting in long-term inhibition (Goldstein et al., 2001; 2005).

2.6 Regulatory issues

The US FDA (www.fda.gov/MedicalDevices/default.htm) recognizes two types of tinnitus treatment devices, hearing aids and tinnitus masker devices (TMD). The later can be used in a variety of forms as wearable devices and appliques for temporary relief. The use of personal music devices for relaxation, as long as no medical claims are made, is unregulated. The FDA defines "a tinnitus masker is an electronic device intended to generate noise of sufficient intensity and bandwidth to mask ringing in the ears or internal head noises. Because the device is able to mask internal noises, it is also used an aid in hearing external noises and speech. TMDs include "in-the-ear" and "behind-the-ear" air conduction configurations. The device type also includes ultrasound TMDs." The FDA treats tinnitus masker devices as Class II with special controls (code KLW) such that the device must meet the FDA recommendations and provide assurances of safety and effectiveness. Specifically there must be a premarket notification that addresses any associated health risks to health and the manufacturer must obtain a substantial equivalence determination from FDA prior to marketing the device. That is what devices on the market are similar to the new device.

The manufacturer may submit a traditional 510(k) or an abbreviated 510(k). An abbreviated 510(k) provides the least burdensome means of demonstrating substantial equivalence for a new device. The abbreviated 510(k) submission must include the proposed labeling for the new device specifying device description, intended use, and directions. Furthermore, information on device development, performance specifications, testing methods, test data and description of the risk analysis used must be furnished. A labeled drawing, similar to that used in a patent and a discussion of the device characteristics related to the risks in a class II special controls device is needed as well as a declaration of conformity to any standard selected adhering to the testing described in the standard.

A traditional 510(k) must meet all of the informational and data requirements of an abbreviated 510(k) including methods, data, acceptance criteria, and conclusions; however the device description is more formal including:

- "a description of the components of the device and its assembly,
- a description of any accessories used with the device,
- the range of dimensions, shapes, and device designs,
- engineering drawings, if applicable,
- a description of the principle of operation (i.e., the scientific principles behind how the device achieves its intended use).

For ultrasound TMDs, engineering drawings should show:

- detailed dimensions of the circular tip area of the transducer that will contact the mastoid area,
- associated static force necessary to achieve output levels, and
- how the static force is achieved."

The safety risks and the mitigations are summarized in Table II. Note that the mitigations are labeling and testing

Generally three predicate devices are selected to show how the new device is both similar to and different from the FDA submitted device. The manufacturers, predicate device names, and 510(k) numbers should accompany the comparative performance comparisons.

Preclinical and clinical studies for traditional 510(k) application can be submitted if needed. FDA recommends a preclinical to evaluate the biocompatibility of device materials contacting patients if it is not already approved. For ultrasound TMDs, a risk analysis of potential ultrasonic energy adverse effects, as tissue heating of tissue or changes in auditory threshold, must be submitted. Maximum output intensity must be measured and reported to avoid cavitation.

Clinical studies are not usually required, but if needed, the following specifications are recommended:

risks	mitigation
• worsening of tinnitus	labeling; clinical testing
• change in hearing	preclinical testing; labeling; clinical testing
• adverse tissue reaction	preclinical testing
• electrical hazards	preclinical testing
• tissue heating (ultrasonics)	preclinical testing
• improper use	labeling

Table 2. The safety risks and the suggest FDA mitigation

- "design, i.e., masking pattern, peak intensity or duration, etc. dissimilar from any design previously cleared under a premarket notification;
- new technology, i.e., technology different from that used in legally marketed TMDs;
- Indications for use dissimilar from TMDs of the same type.'

If a clinical study is carried out it should address issues related to changes in auditory thresholds, pre- and post-exposure to ultrasonic masking stimuli, possible negative side effects of fatigue, headaches, nausea, irritability, and "fullness" in the ear. If a clinical study is needed to demonstrate substantial equivalence, i.e., conducted prior to obtaining 510(k) clearance of the device, the study must be conducted under the Investigational Device Exemptions (IDE) and have institutional review board (IRB) approval with signed and understood, informed consent.

The European Union (EU) assigns medical devices to four groups according to their level of perceived risk before they are approved. Class I is low risk, IIa (tinnitus maskers), IIb (which includes diagnostic radiology equipment) and Class III is high risk (implantable devices). Compliance with the EU guideline leads to CE (conformance mark) certification for medical devices. The method of device development includes specifying performance to specifications, hazard analysis, frequency measurement, function assessment, safety and sustainability must be documentation before applying for the CE mark.

2.7 Innovation in sound therapy

The animal work of (Norena and Eggermont, 2005) indicates that moderate levels of high frequency noise stimulation post noise exposure mitigated the neuroreprograming in the auditory cortex characteristically associated with tinnitus. This is direct substantiation that external sound or masking can alter the neural substrate of tinnitus. Moffat et al., (2009) applied these concepts to humans by fitting tinnitus patients with either standard hearing aids or aids with a broad frequency response to 8 kHz. Neither amplification scheme altered the tinnitus spectrum or its loudness. The most obvious conclusion is there was insufficient high frequency stimulation to alter the tinnitus spectrum. The same conclusion was reached by Schaette et al., (2010) is a similar but not identical study. The issue is not masking since most individuals can experience tinnitus masking.

The critical elements in tinnitus maskers for the purpose of brain therapy are very high frequency stimulation, beyond standard hearing aids, individual adjustability for custom fitting and the ability to affect tinnitus loudness through dedicated use. Treatment of tinnitus with high frequency signals that cover the tinnitus pitch frequencies (areas of hearing loss) and higher has been shown to be effective using behavioral and imaging studies (Shulman et al., 2004; Lanting et al., 2009 for review). The use of the UltraQuiet device with a pass band of 6-20 kHz not only masked the tinnitus but also reduced minimal masking levels by an average of 10 dB (5-25 dB), increased hearing in the tinnitus spectrum by 10 dB and reduced tinnitus severity by questionnaire over a period of eight weeks (Goldstein et al., 2005). Nonetheless, the compliance of patients has been less than expected outside the research laboratory environment unless the device is used in context of counseling and support. There is a need for a home based unit that will provide the time needed to insure therapeutic success, especially in environments lacking audiological infrastructure and /or professional supervision.

2.8 Tinnitus masker for in home use

Bone conduction delivery is employed to provide a comfortable high frequency listening experience. The transducer is a custom-made aluminum ceramic bimorph with a high-frequency limit of 50 kHz. The transducer is coupled to the skin and held in place with a band, much as are traditional clinical bone-conduction transducers. Rather than using synthetic recorded stimuli the sound from a television is the source which is encode by a directional microphone (or direct out port), high passed filtered (4kHz) and amplitude modulated by a variable carrier(s). The carrier can be tuned by the patient (that is selected from ~4 to 20+ kHz) to match their tinnitus and compensate for their skull acoustics by adjusting to "confortable (a mixture of the carrier frequency and idiopathic skull resonances). The carrier can be set to sweep if adjustment is not desired. In the frequency sweep mode the modulated audio sound retains it pitch qualities but varies in loudness as brain/skull resonances are passed by the sweep. The wideband multiplication and a summing analog modulator circuit have easy to use dial-in carrier frequencies. This module outputs to an amplifier and bone conduction transducer (UltraQuiet). All the processing is preengineered in the module (Vicari et al., 2008).

In the first example a sibilant sound /s/ (Figure 1) is modulated by two carriers at 6 and 12 kHz. The amplitude of the 12 kHz carrier is higher by 10 dB to increase salience. An example of speech prior to being filtered and modulated is depicted in the upper panel (A) of Figure 2. After the speech signal is modulated (multiplied) by twin carriers (19 and 22 kHz) the resulting full amplitude modulated signal has an effective band width of 16-24 kHz (panel B). The use of this system will enhance intelligibility (Vicari et al., 2008) but the rationale is to use television as an engaging source for high frequency therapy as well as conventional listening and viewing.

The details of the system are presented in Figure 3. The anticipated source is a television to maintain interest, but it could be a radio, computer or any media device, the signal is fed into a modulator (modified Analog Devices ADL 5319). The carrier(s) is supplied by a modified oscillator chip (Analog Devices AD 5932 generator) with a programmable frequency profile. The carrier can be swept in frequency over the tinnitus spectrum and higher. Alternatively two carriers can be used that are fixed or sweep over more constrained ranges over the same tinnitus spectrum. The carrier frequency shift is not perceived as changes in pitch as much as loudness fluctuations as the carrier interact with head resonances. When the modulating frequency (filtered television signal with a 2-8 kHz pass band) is multiplied by a carrier the result is the carrier plus and minus the modulator. So if the carrier is 12 kHz the resulting signal is 12 $^{+}/_{-}$ 2-8 kHz. The carrier is present in full amplitude Modulation (AM) absent in carrier suppressed modulation (CSM) and absent along with lower sideband in upper sideband modulation (USM). Going forward with the example

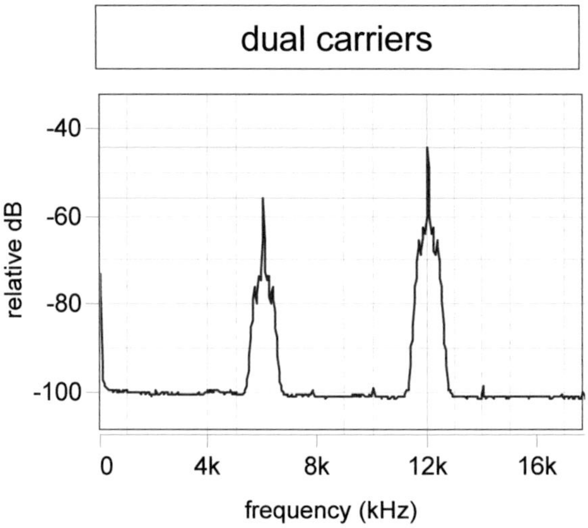

Fig. 1. The double carrier modulation of /s/ is depicted.

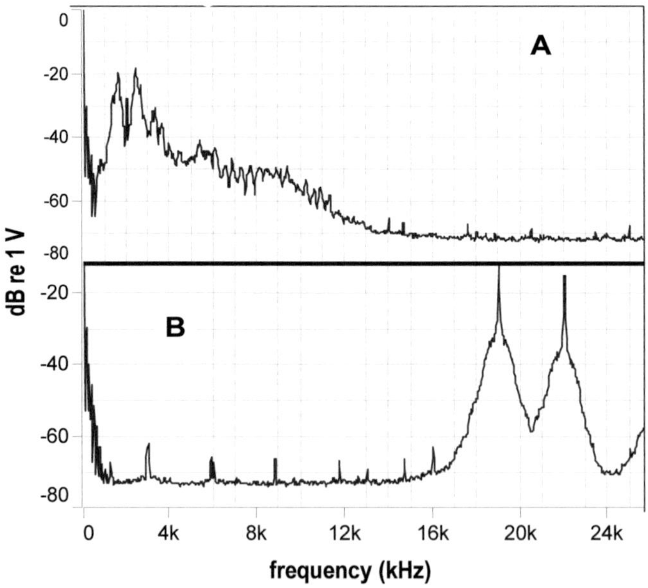

Fig. 2. The speech segment to be modulated is depicted in panel A, and the dual carrier modulation is depicted in panel B. By selecting the appropriate carrier or carriers the high frequency stimulation can be shifted and customized to the patient to treat the tinnitus pitch, spectrum and higher frequency areas as indicated by high frequency audiometry.

of the 12 kHz carrier the USB signal would have a pass band from 14-20 kHz. AM mode is not used for speech perception since the carrier is the strongest signal, usually very audible; resulting in hearing a steady pitch plus the modulated speech. For tinnitus masking, this is not such a problem because the goal is high frequency stimulation. As depicted in Figure 3 (upper panel A) there is an attenuator to adjust the level of high frequency stimulation which should be 12 dB above sensation level (SL). Low level stimulation is important because hyperacusis is always a concern in severe tinnitus. Returning to Figure 3 (B panel) the output of the modulator, appropriately attenuated is amplified and fed into a custom aluminum ceramic transducer. The transducer should be placed on the skin of the head near the ear, the mastoid region is recommended. Alternatively, the transducer can be placed on the skin of the skull in front of the ear, on the so called "ultrasonic window". The maximum output for the FDA approved amplified/transducer is < 76 dB SPL equivalent (maximum force is 100 dB re 1 μN), thus this would be unsuitable for those (ager 18+) with more than a 60 dB HL hearing loss. A newer amplifier has 20 dB more output. The frequency sweep mode may be best if limited audiometric infrastructure is available.

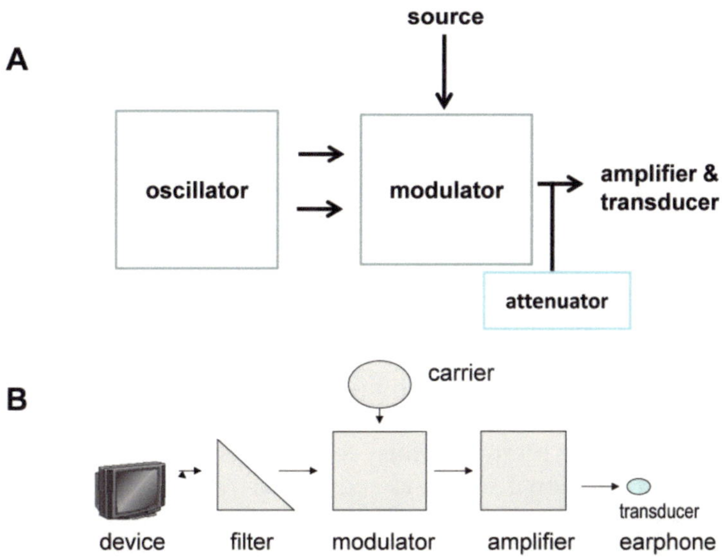

Fig. 3. The home medical device for tinnitus is depicted. The essential elements, oscillator, modulator and amplifier are fed into an UltraQuiet amplifier and transducer after preprocessing a television signal (panel A). The entire system is depicted in panel B.

In reference to the UltraQuiet amplifier and transducer's FDA compliance, the force exerted by bone conduction vibrators in audiometry and its relation to hearing level is normally measured according to standard ANSI S3.43-1992, for frequencies up to 4 kHz. There is no standard for calibration of bone conduction force in the UltraQuiet™ range from 6 kHz to 20 kHz. There are also no artificial mastoids with impedance calibrated in this range. The following measurements use a frequency of 6 kHz, and extrapolate the results to the higher frequencies. Although the standard is given in force, measurements are often made in acceleration for practical reasons, and converted to force (Hakansson et al., 1985). Hakansson et al., in their calibration of direct bone conduction, faced a similar need to extrapolate from existing standards.

The formula for calculation of force is $F = |Z| \times A/\omega$, where: F = force in N, A = acceleration in m/s^2, $|Z|$ = mechanical point impedance in Ns/m, ω = angular frequency (radians/s).
Using the above equation, the following numbers apply to 6 kHz, taken from Table 1 in Hakansson et al. (1985), based on the Reference Equivalent Threshold Force Levels (RETFL) as proposed in ISO/DIS 7566, and the mechanical impedance of the head at the skin surface in the draft revision of IEC publication 373, 1971.

Frequency:	6000 Hz
RETFL (dB re 1 mN):	40.0 dB
Mechanical Impedance (dB re: 1 Ns/$_m$):	34.0 dB
RETAL (dB acceleration re: 1 cm/s^2):	17.5 dB (-2.5 dB re 1 m/s^2)

The measurement system consisted of a Brüel & Kjaer 4374 accelerometer with a Brüel & Kjaer Pulse 3560 analysis system. As reference levels for calibration, a Radioear B-71 bone vibrator was used with its standard headband as the static force (measured at 4.4 N) compared to a plastic headband with a static force of 1.5 N and an Madsen Orbiter 922 audiometer, at 0 dB HL and 55 dB HL, on a live human head, since no artificial mastoids are calibrated in the higher frequency range. There was no difference between the two headbands; with complete coupling, the difference in static force made no difference in the measured acceleration. A simple plastic headband was selected for comfort and appearance.
Based on the above table, using an artificial mastoid, at 0 dB HL and 6 kHz, the force should be 40.0 dB and the acceleration should be -2.5 dB. In the experimental arrangement, the acceleration was –12.5 dB re 1 m/s^2. Thus a correction factor of 10.0 dB must be added to the data to yield measurements comparable to the standard. This is similar to the method used by Hakansson et al. (1985) to arrive at correction factors for direct bone conduction via a screw attached to the skull. In the same experimental arrangement, the 55 dB HL signal from the audiometer produced a 42.0 dB re 1 m/s^2 acceleration (54.5 dB more than the –12.5 dB acceleration at 0 dB HL), confirming the linearity of the system within 0.5 dB.
The minimum recommended use is one hour daily. Effectiveness can be assessed with tinnitus outcome questionnaires to establish a baseline of functioning; these include the tinnitus intensity index, the annoyance index, and the tinnitus severity index (Goldstein et al.,2001; 2004) which can be filled out by home users.
A stand-alone in home use tinnitus device that employs a recreational source of sound (television) minimizes the need to be in proximity to a hearing health care facility for treatment. Further low cost therapy can be delivered without expensive hospital or practice based facilities; all but eliminating multiple office visits. Compliance will likely improve increasing outcomes. One time purchase eliminated the need for third party carriers to fund on going therapy, particularly in population with a disproportionate access to conventional services. The in home UltraQuiet device will not require special training other than some initial familiarization with the device controls and protocol. There is no need for a medical resource environment for its operation.

Tinnitus and hearing loss are military service-related disabilities for which veteran compensation costs are high and expanding with world-wide theaters of operation (Fausti et al., 2009; Veterans Affairs, 2009). Tinnitus can be induced from blast and noise exposure and a recreational used therapy system can be beneficial in recovery. Rehabilitating injured warfighters can increase readiness as well as be a component in total care. Future plans are to develop a wearable UltraQuiet paired with various types personal listening and multimedia devices for tinnitus therapy.

3. Summary

In summary this tinnitus masking system will deliver high frequency bone conduction stimulation without interfering with the television broadcast acoustics, such that patients can watch engaging television programming and receive tinnitus treatment. The innovation is effortless use by embedding the technology into a recreational activity. High frequency bone conduction stimulation was found to be effective in producing residual inhibition (suppression of tinnitus after device is turned off) and reported in 2001 (Goldstein et al.) before the animal studies provided a rational for such treatment. The bioeffect is now known to be more than residual inhibition, but neuroreprogramming in the auditory and limbic systems. There is no effectiveness if the treatment is not carried out. The goal is high frequency treatment that is effective and fully utilized by wedding it to a recreational use, which in turn would translate into improved quality of life for millions globally.

4. Acknowledgment

UltraQuiet is now the property of Ceres Biotechnology LLC, Richmond Virginia 23298-0168.

5. References

Amoodi HA, Mick PT, Shipp DB, Friesen LM, Nedzelski JM, Chen JM, Lin VY. (2011). The effects of unilateral cochlear implantation on the tinnitus handicap inventory and the influence on quality of life. *Laryngoscope*. Jul;121(7):1536-40.

Annual Benefits Report, Fiscal Year 2009. Department of Veterans Affairs, Veterans Benefits Administration. (http://www.vba.va.gov/REPORTS/abr/2009_abr.pdf)

Arndt S, Aschendorff A, Laszig R, Beck R, Schild C, Kroeger S, Ihorst G, Wesarg T. (2011). Comparison of pseudobinaural hearing to real binaural hearing rehabilitation after cochlear implantation in patients with unilateral deafness and tinnitus. *Otology and Neurotology*. Jan;32(1):39-47.

Bredberg G. (1967). The human cochlea during development and aging. *The Journal of Laryngology & Otology*, 81: 739-758.

Del Bo L, Forti S, Ambrosetti U, Costanzo S, Mauro D, Ugazio G, Langguth B, Mancuso A. (2008). Tinnitus aurium in persons with normal hearing: 55 years later. *Otolaryngology Head and Neck Surgery*. Sep;139(3):391-4.

Del Bo L, & Ambrosetti U. (2007). Hearing aids for the treatment of tinnitus. *Progress in Brain Ressearch*. 166:341-5.

Eggermont JJ & Roberts LE. (2004). The neuroscience of tinnitus. *Trends in Neuroscience.* 27:676-682

Erlandsson SI, Hallberg LR, Axelsson A. (1992). Psychological and audiological correlates of perceived tinnitus severity. *Audiology.* 31(3):168-79.

Fausti SA, Wilmington DJ, Gallun FJ, Myers PJ, Henry JA. (2009) Auditory and vestibular dysfunction associated with blast-related traumatic brain injury. *Journal Rehabilitation Research Development.* 46(6):797-810.

Goldstein, B., Shulman, A., Lenhardt, M.L., Richards D.G., Madsen, A., Guinta, R. (2001). Long-term Inhibition of Tinnitus by UltraQuiet™ Therapy: Preliminary Report. *International Tinnitus Journal,* 7, 2, 122-127.

Goldstein BA, Lenhardt M.L. Shulman, A. (2005). Tinnitus improvement with ultra high frequency vibration therapy. *International Tinnitus Journal,* 11,1,14-22.

Goldsteim BA, Shulman A Lenhardt ML (2005). Ultrahigh frequency ultrasonic external acoustic stimulation for tinnitus relief: a method for patient selection, International *Tinnitus Journal.* 11(2): 111-114.

Hakansson B, Tjellstrom A, Rosenhall U. (1985). Acceleration levels at hearing threshold with direct bone conduction vs. conventional bone conduction. *Acta Otolaryngologia;*100:240-252.

Heffner HE & Heffner RS. (1986). Hearing loss in Japanese macaques following bilateral auditory cortex lesions. *Journal of Neurophysiology,* 55, 256-271.

Heffner HE & Heffner RS. (1995) Conditioned avoidance. in Methods in Comparative Psychoacoustics (eds. Klump, G.M. et al.) 79-94 Basel: Birkhauser Verlag.

Heller MF. & Bergman M. Tinnitus aurium in normally hearing persons.(1953) *Annals of Otology, Rhinology and Laryngology* 62:73– 83.

Kitajima K, Kitahara M, Kodama A. Can tinnitus be masked by band erased filtered masker? Masking tinnitus with sounds not covering the tinnitus frequency.(1987). *American Journal of Otology* 8:203-6.

Knobel K.& Sanchez TG. Influence of silence and attention on tinnitus perception.(2008). *Otolaryngology Head and Neck Surgery.* Jan;138(1):18-22.

Lanting CP, de Kleine E, van Dijk P. (2009). Neural activity underlying tinnitus generation: results from PET and fMRI. Hearing Research. Sep;255(1-2):1-13.

LeDoux JE (1990). Information flow from sensation to emotion plasticity in the neural computation of stimulus value. IN M. Gabriel & J. Moore (Eds). "Learning and Computational Neuroscience: Foundations of adaptive networks" (pp3-52). Cambridge, MA; Bradford Books; MIT Press.

Lenhardt ML. (2003). Ultrasonic Hearing in Humans: Applications for Tinnitus Treatment. *International Tinnitus Journal.* 9(2):69-75

Meikle MB, Edlefsen LL, Lay JW. (1999). Suppression of tinnitus by bone conduction of ultrasound. Paper presented at the *Twenty-First Annual Meeting of the Association for Research in Otolaryngology,*St. Petersburg Beach, FL, USA

Moffat G, Adjout K, Gallego S, Thai-Van H, Collet L, Noreña AJ. (2009). Effects of hearing aid fitting on the perceptual characteristics of tinnitus. *Hearing Research.* Aug;254(1-2):82-91.

Moller AR, Moller MB, Yokota M. (1992). Some forms of tinnitus may involve the extralemniscal auditory pathway. *Laryngoscope*, 102,10, 1165-1171.

Møller MB, Møller AR, Jannetta PJ, Jho HD. (1993). Vascular decompression surgery for severe tinnitus: selection criteria and results. *Laryngoscope*. Apr;103(4 Pt 1):421-7.

Noreña AJ, & Eggermont JJ (2005). Enriched acoustic environment after noise trauma reduces hearing loss and prevents cortical map reorganization. *Journal of Neuroscience*, Jan, 25(3):699-705

Pan T, Tyler RS, Ji H, Coelho C, Gehringer AK, Gogel SA. (2009). Changes in the tinnitus handicap questionnaire after cochlear implantation. *American Journal of Audiology*. Dec;18(2):144-51.

Schaette R. & Kempter R. (2010). Predicting tinnitus pitch from patients' audiograms with a computational model for the development of neuronal hyperactivity. *Journal of Neurophysiology*. Jun;101(6):3042-52

Schaette R, König O, Hornig D, Gross M, Kempter R (2010). Acoustic stimulation treatments against tinnitus could be most effective when tinnitus pitch is within the stimulated frequency range. *Hearing Research*. Oct 1;269(1-2):95-101

Shulman A. & Goldstein B. (1996). A final common pathway for tinnitus -Implications for treatment. *International Tinnitus Journal*. 2(2):137-142

Shulman A. (1995). A final common pathway for tinnitus - The medial temporal lobe system. *Internal Tinnitus Journal*.1(2):115-126.

Shulman A, Strashun A.M., Avitable J, Lenhardt M.L. Goldstein BA. (2004). Ultra-High frequency acoustic stimulation and tinnitus control: A Positron Emission Tomography Study. *International Tinnitus Journal*, 10, 2, 113-125.

Shulman, A, Goldstein, B, Strashun AM. (2009) Final Common Pathway for Tinnitus: Theoretical and Clinical Implications of Neuroanatomical Substrates. *International Tinnitus Journal*. 15(1):5-50.

Sweetow RW. & Sabes JH. (2010). Effects of acoustical stimuli delivered through hearing aids on tinnitus. Journal of the American Academy of Audiology. Jul-Aug;21(7):461-73.

Syka J. (2004). Plastic changes in central auditory system after hearing loss, restoration of function and during learning. *Physiological Review*. 82:601-636.

Tucker DA, Phillips SL, Ruth RA, Clayton WA, Royster E, Todd AD. (2005). The effect of silence on tinnitus perception. *Otolaryngology Head and Neck Surgury*. Jan;132(1):20-4.

Vernon JA, & Meikle MB. (2000). Tinnitus masking. In RS Tyler (ed.), Tinnitus Handbook. San Diego: Singular, 2000.

Vernon JA, & Meikle MB. (2003). Masking devices alprazolam treatment for tinnitus. *Otolaryngology Clinics of North America* 36; 307–320.

Vicari J, Slane J, Madsen, AG, Lenhardt, ML. (2008). Increasing the Effective Use of High-Frequency Spectrum Tinnitus Therapy. *International Tinnitus Journal*. 14(2):108-11.

Weisz N, hartmann T, Dohrmann K, Schlee W, Norena A. (2006) High frequency tinnitus without hearing loss does not mean absence of deafferentation, *Hearing Research* 222:108-114

www.fda.gov/MedicalDevices/default.htm

Wienbruch C, Paul I, Weisz N, Elbert T, Roberts LE. (2006). Frequency organization of the 40 Hz auditory steady-state response in normal hearing and in tinnitus. *Neuroimage*. 33: 180-194.

Wilson EC, Schlaug G, Pantev C. (2010). Listening to filtered music as a treatment option for tinnitus: A review. *Music Perception*. Apr 1;27(4):327-330.

9

Bhramari Pranayama and Alternative Treatments of Tinnitus: In Pursuit of the Cure

Sidheshwar Pandey
Trinidad and Tobago Association for the Hearing Impaired, DRETCHI
Trinidad and Tobago,
West Indies

1. Introduction

TINNITUS - a symptom which can have a range of adverse effects for a significant number of people with the result of detrimental impacts on their quality of life. However, tinnitus remains poorly understood and there is no uniformly effective therapy.

This chapter is intended to introduce a novel approach to the management of tinnitus using Bhramari Pranayama (BP). Minimal information on alternative clinical management is provided. The chapter addresses treatment options for patients with tinnitus including pharmachological treatment, surgery, electrical stimulation, transcranial magnetic stimulation, masking therapy, hearing aids, ultra high frequency vibration therapy, Neuromonics tinnitus treatment, sound stimulation therapy during sleep, tinnitus retraining therapy, cognitive behavioural therapy, virtual reality therapy, biofeedback therapy, neurofeedback therapy, as well as research leading to tinnitus management and recommendations for future research.

Although there is no cure for tinnitus, research from around the world probes tinnitus's potential therapies. The intensive work in applying the principles of Bhramari Pranayama is explaining successful tinnitus management (Pandey et al., 2010). The primary goal of this chapter is to provide a therapeutic approach (Bhramari Pranayama) for tinnitus sufferers by helping them overcome the loudness of tinnitus, the psychosocial (inability to participate in leisure activity and work, difficulty in concentration, depression) and also the physical (sleep disturbance, muscle tension) consequences of tinnitus. It is important to note that Bhramari Pranayama can be used in patients with a high degree of severity of tinnitus whereas other therapeutic approaches like masking therapy or sound therapy may not be appropriate in the same conditions. The application of the Bhramari Pranayama concept helps the sufferer to design and implement a program to manage their tinnitus and associated difficulties. The concepts of the limbic system and neural plasticity are also addressed, taking into consideration their association with Bhramari Pranayama.

There are three main components of tinnitus which interact with and influence each other. The first being the *acoustic* component, which is perceived most commonly as an undesirable continuous, high pitched ringing sound. The second aspect of tinnitus is the *attentional* component, and this refers to the degree to which the afflicted person listens to or focuses on the tinnitus. The patient often finds it difficult to concentrate on anything else. The third aspect is the *emotional* component, which is an affective reaction to the tinnitus. This component generally determines the severity of a person's response to tinnitus. There is a hierarchy of reactions ranging from frustration or annoyance in milder cases, to anxiety or depression in more severe cases (Kaltenbach, 2009).

In the mid-1990s, researchers began a series of studies using imaging techniques that have helped change our understanding of the mechanics of tinnitus and potential treatment options for it. There have been two reports about the perception of tinnitus which have been carried out by using imaging techniques. The first study used single photon emission computerized tomography (SPECT), which identified the temporal, frontal and parietal lobes, as well as the amygdala and hippocampus as playing roles in tinnitus perception (Shulman et al., 1995). The second study with positron emission tomography (PET) identified the temporal, parietal areas and subcortical structures (Mirz et al., 1999). Previously, it was generally believed that the tinnitus originated in the ear.

Three zones have been identified where tinnitus is perceived. The prefrontal area in relation to attention and stress, the primary temporal area in relation to hearing and related emotive association with the parietal area, and the limbic system that is composed of different subcortical structures that control emotions, learning, memory and motivated behavior (Lopez-Gonzalez & Esteban-Ortega, 2005).

Evidence from human brain imaging studies confirms the involvement of central structures in tinnitus and points to changes not only in the auditory cortex (Giraud et al., 1999; Lockwood et al., 2001) but also in limbic structures associated with emotion (Lockwood et al., 2001). A recent study described structural alterations in the central nervous system that were detected in tinnitus patients using voxel-based morphometry (VBM); it was found that significant decreases of grey matter in the right inferior colliculus and in the left hippocampus confirmed the important role of the limbic system in the pathophysiology of tinnitus (Landgrebe et al., 2009).

2. Treatment of tinnitus

Even with recent medical advances, no therapy has been found to be uniformly effective in the treatment of tinnitus. However, certain forms of therapy are well defined and are used routinely to treat tinnitus.

2.1 Pharmacological treatment

Various pharmacological therapies have been studied in the treatment of tinnitus. Unfortunately, most studies evaluating the efficacy of these drugs have demonstrated variable success. Currently, no pharmacological agent is specifically administered for tinnitus (Patterson & Balough, 2006). The use of drugs should be considered for tinnitus patients only when sleep disorders, depression, and/or anxiety are reported as significant coexisting conditions (Dobie, 1999). The rationale behind the use of these agents for the treatment of tinnitus should not be overlooked. A consistent approach to studying pharmacological agents in tinnitus is needed.

The use of alternative medication such as magnesium, zinc, melatonin, lidocaine, botulinum toxins, antioxidant minerals, B vitamins, Ginkgo biloba and other herbal remedies have reduced the severity of tinnitus in some sufferers (Fornaro & Martino, 2010).

2.1.1 Ginkgo biloba

Ginkgo biloba extract is a powerful glutamate antagonist which acts as a strong antioxidant within the cochlea, helping to minimize the damage caused by free radical build-up. EGB761 is the most common isolate of Ginkgo biloba which increases body circulation and has benefits for vascular insufficiency and cognitive function (Seidman & Babu, 2003). Improvement in blood circulation to the organ of Corti has been suggested as a mechanism for ameliorating tinnitus (Holgers et al., 1994; Patterson & Balough, 2006). In a rodent model, EGB761 resulted in a statistically significant decrease in the behavioral manifestation of tinnitus induced by sodium salicylate toxicity even at minimal doses (Jastreboff et al., 1997). Some reports indicated that Ginkgo biloba, one of the most ancient medicinal plants, provided significant improvement for tinnitus patients (Coles, 1988). Other contradictory studies have not identified any effect for tinnitus (Ernst & Stevinson, 1999; Drew & Davies, 2001). Holstein (2001) reported that short-standing disorders have a better prognosis and better results can be expected from early-onset treatment. Recent reports showed that Ginkgo biloba extract alone or combined with Bhramari Pranayama have positive effects on tinnitus (Pandey et al., 2010).

2.2 Surgery

Traditional medical approaches to the treatment of tinnitus have included surgical procedures. Surgery may be performed in order to attend to an underlying process or disease which may ultimately influence the tinnitus or more directly, for the specific purpose of tinnitus relief. Surgical treatment of tinnitus includes destructive procedures such as neurectomies, stapedectomies and tympanosympathectomies. Translabyrinthine procedures for the removal of acoustic neuromas and sectioning of the eighth nerve to eliminate vertigo are analogous to cutting the eighth nerve as a surgical intervention for tinnitus (House & Brackmann, 1981).

2.3 Electrical stimulation

A Berlin physician, Dr C. J. C. Grapengeiss (1801) reported on the use of electrical current in suppressing tinnitus. Since then rigorous efforts have been made to evaluate the same treatment. The use of electrical stimulation for the relief of tinnitus has demonstrated some positive findings. However, there is some indication that it may produce damage to the neural tissue particularly with the use of direct current (Hazell et al., 1989; Staller, 1998). Alternating current does not cause these damaging effects but its effectiveness is limited to very few patients. Electrical stimulation is not a method that is presently useful in clinical practice to treat tinnitus but is considered a promising area of investigation. (Dauman, 2000; Rubinstein & Tyler, 2004). Recently, cochlear implants were found to be effective for reducing the sensation of tinnitus (Vernon, 2000; Ruckenstein et al., 2001). Tinnitus is usually masked in patients with cochlear implants. The reorganization of the central auditory nervous system after restoration of peripheral sensory input may have positive effects on tinnitus improvement (Moller, 2003; Del Bo & Ambrosetti, 2007). Cochlear implants have also been observed to exacerbate tinnitus (Tyler, 1995). Cortical electric stimulation of the auditory cortex for treatment of tinnitus is still at the research level (De Ridder et al., 2007a).

2.4 Transcranial magnetic stimulation

Recently it has been shown that stimulation of specific regions of the human brain can alter (suppress) tinnitus in some patients (De Ridder et al., 2004; De Ridder et al., 2006). Auditory cortex stimulation can be performed with a strong impulse of magnetic field that induces an electrical current in the brain (transcranial magnetic stimulation) or with implanted electrodes (De Ridder et al., 2004; De Ridder et al., 2006). There have been a number of recent reports about the possible therapeutic effects of repetitive transcranial magnetic stimulation (rTMS) for the treatment of tinnitus.

Burst rTMS (Repetitive transcranial magnetic stimulation) is capable of suppressing narrowband/white noise tinnitus much better than tonic rTMS (De Ridder et al., 2007b). Burst firing is a more powerful activator of the cerebral cortex than tonic firing (Lisman 1997; Swadlow and Gusev, 2001; Sherman, 2001). This may be related to the fact that burst activation requires less temporal integration to reach the threshold of a neuron and bursts may activate neurons that are not activated by tonic stimulations, unmasking dormant synapses (Moller, 2006).

Mixed findings have been reported when considering the efficacy of rTMS. The results of some studies suggest that rTMS might be a useful treatment for tinnitus (Kleinjung et al., 2008; Khedr et al., 2008; Lopez-Ibor et al., 2008). Lee et al., 2008 did not report statistically significant improvements.

In spite of the many advances in medical science, progress in treatment of tinnitus has been tardy. Thus far, tinnitus remains a condition which is mainly refractory to conventional medical approaches. The uses of medication, electrical suppression, cochlear implants or surgical procedures are potential medical treatments of any underlying aetiological conditions.

Regardless of the form of treatment, sound is used in one way or another to distract attention from the tinnitus and to reduce the brain's perceived need for stimulation (Henry et al., 2002). Traditionally, three general types of treatments have been most commonly used: masking, hearing aids, and sound therapy in combination with counseling. Acoustic therapy involves using an external sound to reduce or eliminate the perception of tinnitus (Folmer & Carroll, 2006; Vernon & Meikle, 2000) or modify the individuals' emotional reaction to it (Davis, 2006). Sound stimulation may also reverse or alter the abnormal cortical reorganisation thought to be responsible for tinnitus (Norena et al., 2008).

2.5 Masking therapy

A Parisian physician, Jean Marie Gaspard Itard, advocated the use of masking in 1801. Masking by various noises was methodically applied as a remedy for tinnitus in 1821 by Itard. In 1883, Urbantschitsch extensively studied masking of tinnitus by pure tones, such as tuning forks. Jones & Knudsen (1928) created the first electrical masking device (Henry, 1992). Masking devices were introduced on the principle of distraction, that is, if a level of noise, usually 'white noise', is introduced, it can reduce the contrast between the tinnitus signal and background activity in the auditory system, causing a decrease in the patient's perception of their tinnitus (Vernon, 1977).

It is important not to confuse the term 'masking', as used in tinnitus masking, with the masking used in audiological testing. In audiometry, masking occurs largely at the level of the cochlea due to interaction of travelling waves of the stimulus and masker (Searchfield et al., 2010). Tinnitus is a neural representation of a sound, not a physical sound wave, and as such masking cannot occur at the level of the cochlea. Instead, tinnitus masking must occur through another central mechanism. This conclusion is supported by many studies showing that masking of tinnitus does not behave like the masking of an external sound (Vernon & Meikle, 2000). In conventional masking, a pure tone cannot successfully mask a broadband sound, but, in tinnitus masking, some studies have found that presentation of a pure tone can mask tinnitus that is perceived as a broadband sound (Vernon & Meikle, 2000; Searchfield et al., 2010).

A variety of masking stimuli have been used for tinnitus relief. The use of a narrowband noise centered around the perceived pitch of the tinnitus is an attempt to provide relief by either completely or partially obscuring the patient's perception of the tinnitus (Vernon, 1977). Narrowband noise was once considered the most common form of acoustic tinnitus management. There are other stimuli now being increasingly recommended (Sweetow & Sabes, 2010). Henry et al. (2004) & Hann et al. (2008) found dynamic sounds, such as music and rain, to be more effective as maskers compared to narrowband and broadband noise.

The complete masking approach used initially, incorporated the increase of intensity or volume to a level where the tinnitus became imperceptible (Coles, 1997). Later research indicated that using low levels of white noise which was barely audible was more effective in achieving adaptation or down regulation (habituation of disordered auditory perception) (Mckinney et al., 1995; Jasterboff, 1995).

2.6 Hearing aids

Hearing aids have been long recognized to reduce the bothersome effects of tinnitus (Saltzman & Ersner, 1947; Surr et al., 1985; Melin et al., 1987). Amplified external sounds or the internal noise of hearing aids could mask the tinnitus (Tyler & Bentler, 1987). Many tinnitus patients with hearing loss have benefited from a hearing aid. Hearing aids help in their hearing disability and also reduce the severity of their tinnitus.

The exact mechanisms underlying the beneficial effects of amplification are uncertain, but it may be that tinnitus is exacerbated by silence, as the brain then seeks out the neural stimulation it is being deprived of by the hearing loss. Amplification increases neural activity and may thus assist in "turning down" the brain's sensitivity control. Another apparent factor is that hearing aids amplify background noise sufficiently to partially mask the tinnitus, or at least reduce its contrast to silence (Sweetow & Henderson, 2010).

2.7 Ultra-high-frequency vibration therapy

Ultraquiet, a new commercial innovation is a high-frequency bone conduction therapy that aims to reduce long term tinnitus severity by delivering amplitude modulated musical type tones in the range of 10-20 kHz. Research by Goldstein et al. (2005) pointed out four underlying mechanisms that contributed to relief: ultra high-frequency masking, residual inhibition, neurological reprogramming and habituation. Sensorineural hearing loss mainly in the higher frequencies is mostly accompanied with high pitched tinnitus (Shulman et al., 1991) and also leads to cortical reprogramming (Engineer et al., 2004; Lee et al., 2004). High-frequency stimulation aims at slowing down and reversing the process of cortical reprogramming, possibly even leading to the restoration of a normal frequency map.

2.8 Neuromonics tinnitus treatment

The Neuromonics Tinnitus Treatment, one of the newer sound-therapy approaches for tinnitus sufferers, uses a portable listening device to deliver a customized acoustic neural stimulus (Davis et al., 2007). The pocket-sized device emits a high-frequency (up to 12,500 Hz) acoustic stimulus that is customized and spectrally modified based on a patient's individual hearing profile. The use of the device in combination with the educational and counseling program is intended to address the three components that together produce the problems most commonly experienced by tinnitus sufferers. These are: (1) audiological (hearing loss often triggers tinnitus), (2) neurological (how the brain responds), and (3) psychological (how people react to tinnitus). The high-frequency stimulation from the device produces an engrossing and enriching acoustic environment for the brain, thereby promoting neural plastic changes that counteract the effects of hearing loss on the tonotopic order in the auditory cortex (Sinopoli et al., 2007).

2.9 Sound stimulation therapy during sleep

Sound stimulation during sleep is one of the new strategies for treating subjective tinnitus. The stimulus is a sound that mimetized the tinnitus and was fixed at the same tinnitus intensity and then applied through an iPod. They proposed that the sound stimulation with the same characteristics in frequency and intensity as the tinnitus is a way of reinstalling the normal balance in the central level processing of information, hypothesizing that tinnitus emerges to replace an input deficit. This technique provides a treatment of tinnitus during sleep without interfering with the patient's daytime activities (Pedemonte et al., 2010).

Hearing aids, tinnitus maskers, and tinnitus instruments may provide relief for a proportion of tinnitus sufferers, however the success rate for each of these forms is not precisely known.

2.10 Tinnitus Retraining Therapy (TRT)

Our brains have the ability to select sounds that are important to us and to ignore those that are not (Jastreboff and Hazell, 1998). If the tinnitus is not important to the patient anymore then the patient should be able to ignore the sound even if it is still there.

TRT is a clinical implementation of the "neurophysiological model" of tinnitus (Jastreboff, 2004; Jastreboff & Hazell, 2004). TRT involves facilitating habituation to the tinnitus signal by a combination of retraining counseling and sound therapy with broadband noise as well as environmental sounds (Han et al., 2009). Patients with more troublesome tinnitus are advised to wear ear-level devices (sound generators, hearing aids, or combination instruments) to optimize the habituation process. These devices ensure a monotonous, low-level sound that reduces the relative strength of the tinnitus neural signal, which presumably makes the tinnitus signal "less detectable" by the brain (Jastreboff & Hazell, 1993). Reduced detection of the tinnitus signal by the brain at subconscious (subcortical) levels is thought to facilitate habituation of tinnitus-induced reactions and subsequently, habituation of tinnitus perception (awareness) at the conscious (cortical) level. The perception of sound can only then be habituated if it does not evoke an emotional response (Jastreboff & Hazell, 1998). Habituation of tinnitus means that the tinnitus-related neuronal activity is blocked from reaching the limbic and autonomic nervous systems and consequently there are no negative reactions to the tinnitus (habituation of reaction). Moreover, the auditory system is capable of blocking this tinnitus-related neuronal activity, preventing it from reaching higher cortical areas and thus being perceived (habituation of perception) (Jastreboff, P.J. & Hazell, J.W, 2006). Recognition of the importance of the contributory effects of the limbic and autonomic nervous systems is a major aspect of this treatment model. The long term impact of TRT is limited (Dobie, 1999) and it can take up to one to two years to observe stable effects. It has also been noted that there is a need for better experimental designs in the studies on TRT efficacy (Wilson et al., 1998; Kroener-Herwig et al., 2000).

Psychological forms of treatment for tinnitus have included progressive muscular relaxation training, biofeedback, hypnosis, and cognitive-behavioral intervention (Sweetow, 2000; Henry & Wilson, 2000). These types of therapy are not intended to remove or reduce the perceived tinnitus in any way, but help the patient to better cope with tinnitus.

2.11 Cognitive Behavioral Therapy (CBT)

The patient who is severely disturbed by tinnitus can be described as having additional emotional problems, such as depression or anxiety disorder. Treatment of these emotional problems, along with helping the patient to learn better coping strategies can often help the patient deal with their tinnitus (House, 1997). CBT is one of the psychological therapies that have been utilized in the treatment of tinnitus. It is a behavioral counseling technique designed to modify a person's emotional reaction to tinnitus. The goal of CBT in tinnitus treatment is to first recognize and then correct any maladaptive thought patterns about tinnitus (Tyler, 2006). The objective is to desensitize the individuals so that they can accept its presence and still choose to ignore it. The tinnitus sound is still there, however, it is the way in which the patient thinks about the tinnitus that results in specific reactions (Henry & Wilson, 2001). Studies have demonstrated that CBT helped patients reduce tinnitus related distress (Zachriat & Kroner-Herwig, 2004). However, not all patients require a major emphasis on cognitive behavioral therapy.

2.12 Virtual reality therapy

Following the analogy of CBT, the purpose is to act on the sub-cortical mechanisms of integration, thus allowing the patient to willingly manipulate the tinnitus in a visual and auditory 3-Dimensional (3D) virtual environment to control or "master" tinnitus (Londero et al., 2010). The application is based on the model of visual virtual reality coupled with accurate auditory spatial image, as well as a natural sensorimotor interaction provided through the use of two elements. The overall procedure consists of, in the first place, the creation of an auditory avatar (auditory image of patient's tinnitus), and secondly, the inclusion of an interactive auditory–visual virtual environment where the different audio components are spatialized according to the navigation and manipulation of the patient. Londero et al. (2010) believed that immersion in virtual reality can contribute to tinnitus treatment by promoting plasticity, through the active manipulation of a 3D auditory object linked to a visual representation.

Unilateral subjective tinnitus sufferers have the opportunity to voluntarily manipulate an auditory and visual image of their tinnitus (tinnitus avatar) in auditory and visual 3D virtual reality environments. In practice, the patients would be able to convert their subjective auditory perception of the tinnitus avatar and to have the advantage of the multimodal virtual awareness they experience in hearing, seeing and spatial control. Repeated sessions of such virtual reality immersions are then supposed to contribute to tinnitus treatment by promoting cerebral plasticity. Further, clinical research is necessary to demonstrate the clinical relevance in alleviating tinnitus.

2.13 Biofeedback therapy

Biofeedback is a relaxation technique which allows the patient to control certain autonomic bodily functions such as muscle tension, pulse and level of brain activity. The application of biofeedback technique in tinnitus management was first reported by House & colleagues in

1977. With the use of biofeedback, the patient learns to gain control of certain physiologic functions of his/her body with the help of a device that displays the results of this physiologic function electronically (Grossan, 1976). It is designed to train the patient in relaxation procedures that may help him/her to control his/her stress level and ultimately the tinnitus (Shulman, 1997). Biofeedback can help patients suffering from tinnitus, especially during rest (Podoshin et al., 1995). Electromyogram (EMG) activity is used to observe how relaxation techniques effect muscle relaxation. Treatment of tinnitus by EMG biofeedback is most effective (Podoshin et al., 1995). Studies have shown some promise in the relief of tinnitus from these techniques (House, 1978; White et al., 1986; Newman et al., 1997).

2.14 Neurofeedback therapy

Neurofeedback is a recent development in which brain waves are observed. The main categories of brain waves are Beta (awake), Alpha (calm relaxation), Theta (light sleep) and Delta (deep sleep). Neurofeedback is a form of biofeedback related to aspects of the electrical activity of the brain such as frequency, location or amplitude of specific EEG activity. Neurofeedback is a computerized learning strategy that enables people to voluntarily alter their own brain activity. Chronic tinnitus sufferers have different patterns of brain activity compared with those with normal hearing (Weisz et al., 2005). Many individuals with tinnitus have abnormal oscillatory brain activity. This pathological activity can be normalized by neurofeedback techniques (Weisz et al., 2005). This is achieved mainly through enhancement of tau activity (8-12 Hz activity as tau activity).

The brains of tinnitus sufferers showed that reduced Alpha power (8-12 Hz) and enhancement in the Delta (1.5-4 Hz) and gamma power (>30 Hz) brainwave range. These differences were especially pronounced in the brain's temporal cortical regions. Delta enhancement and Alpha reduction were strongly correlated with tinnitus-related distress variables with a focus on the right temporal and also left frontal cortex. The right temporal and left frontal cortex might be involved in a tinnitus-related cortical network, in which the temporal region is associated more with perceptual issues (aspects concerning the character of the sound, e.g., tonal or noise-like, loudness), and the left frontal region more with affective distress and motivational attention of tinnitus (the tinnitus becoming a signal of high importance, so that it draws the attention of the individual) (Weisz et al., 2005). A temporarily generated tau rhythm (8–12 Hz) and slow waves in the Delta range (3–4 Hz) have been used as a neurofeedback protocol to treat tinnitus. In other words, boosting Alpha frequencies and cutting Delta activity using neurofeedback have shown some success in reducing tinnitus (Crocetti et al., 2011). It has also been reported that the use of neurofeedback therapy to manipulate cortical networks can be helpful in reducing tinnitus loudness and distress (Schlee et al., 2008).

2.15 Bhramari Pranayama

Yoga, an ancient philosophy and practice undertaken as a path towards self-realisation, was originated in India in at least 1000 B.C. (Feuerstein, 1990). The beginnings of yoga have been traced to India's oldest sacred text, the *Rig-Veda* (Iyengar, 1991, 1996; Feuerstein, 2003). The word 'yoga' comes from the sanskrit word '*yuj*', which means to join or integrate, to make whole, to connect, or to unite (Iyengar, 1991, 1966; Feuerstein, 2003). A yogic technique, Pranayama, is a method of controlling "*prana*" or life force through the regulation of breathing. It is the breathing process or control of the motion of inhalation, exhalation and the retention of the vital energy. Pranayama is an important aspect of yoga that deals with the connection between breathing patterns and emotional states (Fried, 1993). These techniques aim at reducing anxiety levels in individuals, increasing parasympathetic activity in the milieu of the autonomic nervous system and at times actually inducing great muscular stretching through specific body postures. A breathing technique in pranayama is used to control, improve or refine the breathing processes, thereby energizing the body and calming the mind (Samskriti & Franks, 1978). Paroxysmal Gamma brain waves produced during the Bhramari Pranayama (Vialatte et al., 2009) which is associated with positive thoughts, feelings of happiness and acts as a natural antidepressant. The Bhramari Pranayama is one such ancient 'Yogic' breathing exercise that not only includes a unique breathing technique, but also entails placing the body in a relaxing posture with simultaneous generation of a constant humming sound during the phase of expiration. The sound generated in BP is akin to the humming of a bumble bee (Ramdev, 2005). The individual also actively concentrates his/her mind (mindfulness) at the centre of the forehead while closing both ears using the thumbs and placing light pressure on the eyes using the fingers of each hand respectively. Though practice of Bhramari Pranayama has been advocated and documented for its benefits in combating situations like hypertension, insomnia and related anxiety states, its use as a self-induced sound therapy for treating tinnitus has rarely been reported (Pandey et al., 2010). Application of BP has been demonstrated to provide significant levels of relief in tinnitus.

In BP, pressing of the eyeballs leads to stimulation of the vagus nerve which in turn leads to activation of the parasympathetic nervous system (PNS). PNS is associated with a relaxed and calm state of mind and body (Speciale and Stahlbrodt, 1999; Zabara, 1992). Under the relaxing effects of PNS, autonomic nervous system facilitates to decrease the stressing effects of sympathetic nervous system and channels it towards more relaxed PNS. The neuronal reorganization or flexibility can be achieved by duplicating the activity across synapses (Hormuzdi et al., 2004). Repetitive and simultaneous activity of the parasympathetic system during the therapy sessions reduces sympathetic activity in the person and alleviates the anxiety and stress associated with the onset of an attack or the range of distress experienced during the acute tinnitus attack. Reorganization or rearrangement of neural synapses (plasticity) is depicted by the direct correlation observed in the activation of PNS and the reduction of tinnitus and its associated negative emotions (Alkadhi et al., 2005).

It is important to note that BP works as a self-induced sound therapy and is not only a mode to treat tinnitus but also, ocular compression as a part of BP addresses negative association in the limbic system via stimulation of the vagus nerve. There is also a third reason why BP is particularly important, as breathing is very closely related to the activation of the autonomic nervous system (Ballentine, 1976; Hirai, 1975; Brena, 1971). Slower, deeper and more regular breathing is associated with parasympathetic activation effectively leading to a condition described as calm and composed. Yogic breathing exercises can produce beneficial changes in emotional state (Harvey, 1983). BP employs a combination of acoustic therapies to produce a reduction in central nervous system accomplished by stimulating the auditory cortex for tinnitus relief, and to further stimulate parasympathetic nervous system, thus promoting a less negative emotional response.

It is reported that BP not only suppresses the sound of tinnitus, but it also effectively reduces the irritation and annoyance caused by the sound in tinnitus patients. BP has an advantage in cost effectiveness, as there is no maintenance of any kind of devices such as tinnitus maskers, Walkman mini stereo systems and tinnitus instruments. Such practice of Bhramari Pranayama is quiet safe.

In the presence of various approaches for management of tinnitus, none of the traditional approaches have proved to be a universally superior. Indeed, it is generally accepted that no single technique proves to be effective in all cases. However, the combined therapeutic approach (consisting of Bhramari Pranayama, masking therapy and a herbal drug) has significant effects in the management of tinnitus (Pandey et al., 2010).

3. Conclusion

The answer to whether there is a cure for tinnitus may lie in the question itself. Tinnitus may help us in attempting to understand and reveal normal auditory perception. In a study conducted by Del Bo et al. (2008) people with normal hearing experienced tinnitus when kept in a sound proof chamber for 5-10 minutes. Therefore it can be said that the brain abhors silence and resorts to different mechanisms such as release from inhibition in absence of auditory input.

It is difficult to study and treat tinnitus because of the lack of objective tools to quantify and measure it, and as much as the symptoms vary, so does the treatment. There is no one answer for tinnitus treatment for all individuals, though single isolated effects for different individuals are reported. It is now evident that most forms of tinnitus are caused by changes in the function of the central auditory nervous system while these changes are not associated with any detectable anatomical lesion. The tinnitus may be the result of the expression of neural plasticity and anomalies may develop because of reduced input from the ear, lack of sound stimulation, overstimulation or as yet undetermined factors (Jastreboff, 1990). Many individuals have somatic tinnitus where movements of the eyes, head, neck, jaw and shoulder can change the loudness and pitch of their tinnitus. These findings may suggest the involvement of non-auditory centres in the pathogenesis and regulation of tinnitus. Recent advances in the imaging techniques have served to identify the aberrant neural activity that is associated with tinnitus perception. There is mounting evidence from functional neuroimaging studies that abnormal functioning (neuroplastic alterations) of the central nervous system is involved in the pathophysiology of chronic tinnitus (Eichhammer et al., 2007; Smits et al., 2007). Electrophysiological studies have shown a firing rate increase and neuronal synchrony associated with reduced Alpha and enhanced Gamma activity within primary and secondary auditory cortices that could be correlated to tinnitus-related psychological distress (Weisz et al., 2007). Recently, voxel-based morphometry (VBM) has been proposed for the identification of brain areas that display structural changes in tinnitus. A common genetic cause of tinnitus and depression is believed to be a serotonin transporter gene SLC6A4 and is reported as a potential candidate gene (Tyler RS, Coelho C, Noble W., 2006).

Patients with tinnitus present a variety of symptoms, and as a consequence, wide ranges of therapies are available for treatment. Although many of these therapies are effective when applied to individual patients, no study has yet been able to confirm one. Most successful management programs employ multimodal strategies designed to address the specific needs of each patient. A recent study described combined therapy (Bhramari Pranayama, Masking therapy and Ginkgo biloba) as being advantageous in treating patients with tinnitus. Applications of electrical stimulation of the ear through cochlear implants, stimulation to the vagus nerve and specific parts of the brain are already being investigated for the treatment of tinnitus. Ocular compression in Bhramari pranayama has already been explained in the use of vagus nerve stimulation and the limbic system (Pandey et al., 2010). A continued effort coupled with ongoing research is needed to address the questions. A future goal will be to reach the consensus both for patient assessments and for outcome measurements.

4. References

Alkadhi, K. A.; Alzoubi, K. H. & Aleisa, A. H. (2005). Plasticity of synaptic transmission in autonomic ganglia. *Progress in Neurobiology*. Vol.75, No.2, (February 2005), pp.83 - 108, ISSN 0301-0082

Ballentine, R. M. Jr. (1976). The anatomy and physiology of breathing. In: *The Science of Breath,* R. M. Ballentine Jr., (Ed.), Himalayan Institute, ISBN 0893890200, Glenview, IL

Brena, S. F. (1971). *Yoga and Medicine,* Julian Press, ISBN 0140216510, New York

Coles, R. (1998). Trial of an extract of Ginkgo biloba (EGB) for tinnitus and hearing loss. *Clinical Otolaryngology and Allied Sciences,* Vol.13, No.6, (December 1998), pp. 501–2, ISSN 0307-7772

Coles, R. R. (1997). Tinnitus. In: *Scott-Brown's Otolaryngology - Adult Audiology,* 6th Edition, Volume 2, Dafydd Stephens, Chapter 18, Butterworth Heinemann, 0 7506 0596 0, London

Crocetti, A.; Forti, S. & Del Bo, L. (2011). Neurofeedback for subjective tinnitus patients. *Auris Nasus Larynx,* Vol.38, No.6, (May 2011), pp. 735-738, ISSN 0385-8146

Dauman, R. (2000). Electrical stimulation for tinnitus suppression. In: *Tinnitus handbook,* R. Tyler, (Ed.), 377–398, Singular Publishing Group, ISBN 1-56593-922-0, San Diego (CA)

Davis, P. B. (2006). Music and the acoustic desensitization protocol for tinnitus. In: *Tinnitus treatment: Clinical protocols,* R. S. Tyler, (Ed.), 146–160, Thieme, ISBN 1-58890-181-5, New York

Davis, P.; Paki, B. & Hanley, P. (2007). Neuromonics tinnitus treatment. *Ear and Hearing,* Vol.28, No.2, (April 2007), pp. 242-59, ISSN 0196-0202

De Ridder, D.; De Mulder, G.; Verstraeten, E.; Van Der, K. K.; Sunaert, S.; Smits, M.; Kovacs, S.; Verlooy, J.; Van De, H. P. & Moller, A. R. (2006). Primary and secondary auditory cortex stimulation for intractable tinnitus. *ORL Journal for Oto-rhino-laryngology and its related specialties,* Vol.68, No.1, (March 2006), pp. 48-54, ISSN 0301-1569

De Ridder, D.; De Mulder, G.; Walsh, V.; Muggleton, N.; Sunaert, S. & Moller, A. (2004) Magnetic and electrical stimulation of the auditory cortex for intractable tinnitus. Case report. *Journal of Neurosurgery,* Vol.100, No.3, (March 2004) pp.560-564, ISSN 0022-3085

De Ridder, D.; De Mulder, G; Menovsky, T.; Sunaert, S. & Kovacs, S. (2007a). Electrical stimulation of auditory and somatosensory cortices for treatment of tinnitus and pain. *Progress in Brain Research,* Vol.166, (October 2007a), pp. 377-388, ISSN 0079-6123

De Ridder, D.; Van der, L. E..; Van der, K. K.; Menovsky, T.; Van de, H. P. & Moller, A. (2007b). Theta, alpha and beta burst transcranial magnetic stimulation: brain modulation in tinnitus. *International Journal of Medical Sciences,* Vol.4, No.5, (October, 2007b), pp. 237-241, ISSN 1449-1907

Del Bo, L. & Ambrosetti, U. (2007). Hearing aids for the treatment of tinnitus. *Progress in Brain Research,* Vol.166, (October 2007), pp. 341-345, ISSN 0079-6123

Del Bo, L.; Forti, S.; Ambrosetti, U.; Costanzo, S.; Mauro, D.; Ugazio, G.; Langguth, B. & Mancuso, A. (2008). Tinnitus aurium in persons with normal hearing: 55 years later. *Otolaryngology – Head and Neck Surgery.* Vol.139, No.3, (September 2008), pp. 391–394, ISSN 0194-5998

Dobie, R. A. (1999). A review of randomized clinical trials in tinnitus. *The Laryngoscope,* Vol.109, No.8, (August 1999), pp.1202–1211, ISSN 1531-4995

Drew, S. & Davies, E. (2001). Effectiveness of Ginkgo biloba in treating tinnitus: double blind, placebo controlled trial. *British Medical Journal,* Vol.322, No.7278, (January 2001), pp. 73-78, ISSN 0959-8138

Eichhammer, P.; Hajak. G.; Kleinjung, T.; Landgrebe, M. & Langguth, B. (2007). Functional imaging of chronic tinnitus: the use of positron emission tomography. *Progress in Brain Research,* Vol.166, (October 2007), pp.83–88, ISSN 0079-6123

Engineer ND, Percaccio CR, Pandya PK, Moucha, R.; Rathbun, D. L. & Kilgard, M. P. (2004). Environmental enrichment improves response strength, threshold, selectivity, and latency of auditory cortex neurons. *Journal of Neurophysiology,* Vol.92, No.1, (July 2004), pp. 73–82, ISSN 0022-3077

Ernst, E. & Stevinson, C. (1999). Ginkgo biloba for tinnitus: a review. *Clinical Otolaryngology and Allied Sciences,* Vol.24, No.3, (June 1999), pp.164–167, ISSN 0307-7772

Feuerstein, G. (1990). *Yoga: The technology of ecstasy,* The Aquarian Press, ISBN 1852740884, Wellingborough

Feuerstein, G. (2003). *The Deeper Dimension of Yoga: Theory and Practice,* Shambhala, ISBN 9781570629358, Boston

Folmer, R. L. & Carroll, J. R. (2006). Long-term effectiveness of ear-level devices for tinnitus. *Otolaryngology - Head & Neck Surgery,* Vol.134, No.1, (January 2006), pp. 132-137, ISSN 0194-5998

Fornaro, M. & Martino, M. (2010). Tinnitus psychopharmacology: A comprehensive review of its pathomechanisms and management. *Neuropsychiatric Disease and Treatment,* Vol.6, No. 1, (June 2010), pp. 209–218, ISSN 1178-2021

Fried, R. (1993). *The psychology and physiology of breathing,* Plenum Press, ISBN 0306442787, New York

Giraud, A. L.; Chery-Croze, S.; Fischer, G.; Fischer, C.; Vighetto, A.; Grégoire, M. C.; Lavenne, F. & Collet, L. (1999). A selective imaging of tinnitus. *NeuroReport,* Vol.10, No.1, (January 1999), pp. 1–5, ISSN 0959-4965.

Goldstein, B. A.; Lenhardt, M. L. & Shulman, A. (2005). Tinnitus Improvement with Ultra-High-Frequency Vibration Therapy. *International Tinnitus Journal,* Vol. 11, No. 1, (March 2005), pp. 14–22, ISSN 0946-5448

Grossan, M. (1976). Treatment of subjective tinnitus with biofeedback. *Ear Nose Throat Journal,* Vol.55, No.10, (October 1976), pp. 314-318, ISSN 0145-5613.

Han, B. I.; Lee, H.W.; Kim, T.Y.; Lim, J.S. & Shin, K.S. (2009). Tinnitus: characteristics, causes, mechanisms, and treatments. *Journal of Clinical Neurology,* Vol.5, No.1, (March 2009), pp.11-19, ISSN 1738-6586

Hann, D.; Searchfield, G.D.; Sanders, M. & Wise, K. (2008). Strategies for the Selection of Music in the Short-term Management of Mild Tinnitus. *Australian and New Zealand Journal of Audiology*, Vol.30, No.2, (November 2008), pp. 129-140, ISSN 1443-4873

Harvey, J. R. (1983). The effect of yogic breathing exercises on mood. *Journal of the American Society of Psychosomatic Dentistry & Medicine*, Vol.30, No.2, pp. 39-48, ISSN 0003-1194

Hazell, J. W.; Meerton, L. E. & Ryan, R. (1989). Electrical tinnitus suppression. *Hearing Journal*. Vol. 42, pp. 26–33, ISSN 0745-7472

Henry, J. A.; Rheinsburg, B. & Zaugg, T. (2004). Comparison of custom sounds for achieving tinnitus relief. *Journal of the American Academy of Audiology*, Vol.15, No.8, (September 2004), pp. 585-98, ISSN 1050-0545

Henry, J. A.; Schechter, M. A.; Nagler, S. M. & Fausti, S. A. (2002). Comparison of tinnitus masking and tinnitus retraining therapy. *Journal of the American Academy of Audiology*, Vol.13, No.10, (December 2002), pp. 559–581, ISSN 1050-0545

Henry, J. L. & Wilson. P. H. (2000). *The psychological management of chronic tinnitus*, Allyn & Bacon, ISBN 0205313655, Needham Heights (MA)

Henry, J. L. (1992). The Psychological Management of Chronic Tinnitus: An Evaluation of Cognitive Interventions. *Unpublished Thesis*, Vol.1, pp. 49-50, the University of Sydney

Henry, J.L., Wilson, P.H. (2001) The Psychological Management of Chronic Tinnitus: A cognitive-Behavioral Approach. Boston: Allyn & Bacon. In: *Tinnitus treatment, clinical protocols*, R.S. Tyler, (Ed.), Thieme 2005, ISBN 1588901815, New York

Hirai, T. (1975). *Zen Meditation Therapy*, Komiyama, ISBN 0870403486, Tokyo

Holgers, K. M.; Axelsson, A. & Pringle, I. (1994). Ginkgo biloba extract for the treatment of tinnitus. *Audiology*, Vol.33, No. 2, (April 1994), pp. 85–92, ISSN 1735-1936

Holstein, N. (2001). Ginkgo special extract EGb 761 in tinnitus therapy. An overview of results of completed clinical trials. *Fortschr Med Orig*, Vol.118, No.4, (January 2001), pp. 157-64,

Hormuzdi, S. G.; Filippov, M. A.; Mitropoulou, G.; Monyer, H. & Bruzzone, R. (2004). Electrical synapses: a dynamic signalling system that shapes the activity of neuronal networks. *Biochimica et Biophysica Acta*, Vol.1662, No.1-2, (March 2004), pp. 113 - 137, ISSN 0006-3002

House, J. W. & Brackmann, D. E. (1981). Tinnitus: surgical treatment. *Ciba Foundation Symposium*. Vol. 85, pp.204-16, ISSN 0300-5208

House, J. W.; Miller, L. & House, P. R. (1977). Severe tinnitus: treatment with biofeedback training (Results in 41 cases). *Transactions. Section on Otolaryngology. American Academy of Ophthalmology and Otolaryngology*, Vol.84, No.4, (August 1977), pp. 697-703, ISSN 0161-696X

House, J.W. (1978). Treatment of severe tinnitus with biofeedback training. *The Laryngoscope*, Vol.88, No.3, (March, 1978), pp. 406-412, ISSN 1531-4995

House, P.R. (1997). Psychological issues of tinnitus. In: *Tinnitus: diagnosis/treatment*, A. Shulman; J. Aran; J. Tonndorf; H. Feldman & J.A. Vernon, (Eds.), 533-543, Singular Publishing Group, ISBN 1565939611, San Diego

Iyengar, B.K.S. (1991, 1996). *Light on Yoga*, Harper Collins Publishers, ISBN 9780007107001, London

Jastreboff, J.P. & Hazell, J.W.P. (1998). Treatment of tinnitus based in a neurophysiological model. In: *Tinnitus: Treatment and relief*, J. A. Vernon, (Ed.), 201-217, Allyn & Bacon, ISBN 0-205-05929-5, Needham Heights, Massachusetts

Jastreboff, P. J. (1990), Phantom auditory perception (tinnitus): mechanisms of generation and perception. *Neuroscience Research*, Vol.8, No.4, (August 1990), pp. 221-54, ISSN 0168-0102

Jastreboff, P. J. (1995). Processing of the tinnitus signal within the brain. *Proceedings of the Fifth International Tinnitus Seminar*, pp. 498-499, OCLC 36830029, Portland, Oregon, USA, American Tinnitus Association, July 12-15, 1995

Jastreboff, P. J. (2004). The neurophysiological model of tinnitus. In: *Tinnitus: Theory and management*, J.B. Snow, (Ed.), 96–107, BC Decker, ISBN 155009243X, Hamilton (ON)

Jastreboff, P. J., Hazell, J. W. (2004). *Tinnitus retraining therapy: Implementing the neurophysiological model.* Cambridge University Press, ISBN 0521592569, New York

Jastreboff, P. J.; Zhou, S.; Jastreboff, M. M.; Kwapisz, U. & Gryczynska, U. (1997). Attenuation of salicylate-induced tinnitus by Ginkgo biloba extract in rats. *Audiology and Neurotology*, Vol. 2, No. 4, (August 1997), pp. 197–212, ISSN 1420-3030

Jastreboff, P.J. & Hazell, J.W (2006). The neurophysiological model of tinnitus and decreased sound tolerence, In: *Tinnitus treatment: Clinical protocols*, R. S. Tyler, (Ed.), 32-36, Thieme, ISBN 1-58890-181-5, New York

Jastreboff, P.J. & Hazell, J.W. (1993). A neurophysiological approach to tinnitus: clinical implications. *British Journal of Audiology*, Vol.27, No.1, (February 1993), pp. 7–17, ISSN 0300-5364

Kaltenbach, J. A. (2009). Insights on the origins of tinnitus: An overview of recent research. *The Hearing Journal, Vol.* 62, No.2, (February 2009), pp. 26-29, ISSN 0745-7472

Khedr, E. M.; Rothwell, J. C.; Ahmed, M.A. & El-Atar, A. (2008). Effect of daily repetitive transcranial magnetic stimulation for treatment of tinnitus: comparison of different stimulus frequencies. *Journal of Neurology, Neurosurgery & Psychiatry*, Vol.79, No.2, (February 2008), pp. 212-215, ISSN 0022-3050

Kleinjung, T.; Eichhammer, P.; Landgrebe, M.; Sand, P.; Hajak, G.; Steffens, T.; Strutz, J. & Langguth, B. (2008). Combined temporal and prefrontal transcranial magnetic stimulation for tinnitus treatment: a pilot study. *Otolaryngology - Head & Neck Surgery*, Vol.138, No.4, (April 2008), pp. 497-501, ISSN 0194-5998

Kroener-Herwig, B.; Biesinger, E.; Gerhards, F.; Goebel, G.; Greimel, K.V. & Hiller, W. (2000). Retraining therapy for chronic tinnitus: A critical analysis of its status. *Scandinavian Audiology*, Vol.29, No.2, (May 2000), pp. 67-78, ISSN 0105-0397

Landgrebe, M.; Langguth, B.; Rosengarth, K.; Braun, S.; Koch. A.; Kleinjung, T.; May, A.; De Ridder, D. & Hajak, G. (2009). Structural brain changes in tinnitus: grey matter decrease in auditory and nonauditory brain areas. *NeuroImage*, Vol.46, No.1, (May 2009), pp. 213-218, ISSN 1053-8119

Lee, C. C.; Schreiner, C. E.; Imaizumi, K. & Winer, J. A. (2004). Tonotopic and heterotopic projection systems in physiologically defined auditory cortex. *Neuroscience*, Vol.128, No.4, (September 2004), pp. 871–887, ISSN 0306-4522

Lee, S. L.; Abraham, M.; Cacace, A.T. & Silver, S. M. (2008). Repetitive transcranial magnetic stimulation in veterans with debilitating tinnitus: a pilot study. *Otolaryngology - Head & Neck Surgery*, Vol.138, No. 3, (March 2008) pp. 398-399, ISSN 0194-5998

Lisman, J. E. (1997). Bursts as a unit of neural information: making unreliable synapses reliable. *Trends in Neurosciences,* Vol.20, No.1, (January 1997), pp. 38-43, ISSN 0166-2236

Lockwood, A. H.; Wack, D. S.; Burkard, R. F.; Coad, M. L.; Reyes, S. A.; Arnold, S. A. & Salvi, R. J. (2001). The functional anatomy of gaze-evoked tinnitus and sustained lateral gaze. *Neurology,* Vol.56, No.4, (February 2001), pp. 472–480, ISSN 0028-3878

Londero, A.; Viaud-Delmon, I.; Baskind, A.; Delerue, O.; Bertet, S.; Bonfils, P. & Warusfel, O. (2010). Auditory and visual 3D virtual reality therapy for chronic subjective tinnitus: theoretical framework. *Virtual Reality,* Vol.14, No.2, (June 2010), pp. 143-151, ISSN 1359-4338

Lopez-Gonzalez, M. A. & Esteban-Ortega, F. (2005). Tinnitus dopaminergic pathway. Ear noises treatment by dopamine modulation. *Medical Hypotheses,* Vol.65, No. 2, (August 2005), pp. 349–352, ISSN 0306-9877

Lopez-Ibor, J.J.; Lopez-Ibor, M.I. & Pastrana, J.I. (2008). Transcranial magnetic stimulation. *Current Opinion in Psychiatry,* Vol.21, No.6, (November 2008), pp. 640-644, ISSN 09517367

McKinney, C. J.; Hazell, J. W. P. & Graham, R. L. (1995). Retraining therapy -outcome measures. *Proceedings of the Fifth International Tinnitus Seminar,* pp. 498-499, OCLC 36830029, Portland, Oregon, USA, American Tinnitus Association, July 12-15, 1995

Melin, L.; Scott, B.; Lindberg, P. & Lyttkens, L. (1987). Hearing aids and tinnitus—an experimental group study. British Journal of Audiology. Vol.21, No.2, (May 1987), pp. 91–97, ISSN 0300-5364

Mirz, F.; Pedersen, C.B.; Ishizu, K.; Johannsen, P.; Ovesen, T.; Jorgensen, H.S. & Gjedde, A. (1999). Positron emission tomography of cortical centers of tinnitus. *Hearing Research,* Vol.134, No.1, n.d., pp.133– 44, ISSN 0378-5955

Moller, A. (2006). *Neural plasticity and disorders of the nervous system.* Cambridge University Press, ISBN 0521846676, Cambridge

Moller, A. R. (2003). Pathophysiology of tinnitus. *Otolaryngologic Clinics of North America,* Vol. 36, No.2, (April, 2003), pp. 249-66, ISSN 0030-6665

Newman, C.W.; Warton, J.A. & Jacobson, G.P. (1997). Self-focused and somatic attention in patients with tinnitus. *Journal of the American Academy of Audiology,* Vol.8, No.3, (June 1997), pp. 143-149, ISSN 1050-0545

Norena, A. J.; Gourevitch, B.; Pienkowski, M.; Shaw, G. & Eggermont, J. J. (2008). Increasing spectrotemporal sound density reveals an octave-based organization in cat primary auditory cortex. *The Journal of Neuroscience,* Vol.28, No.36, (September 2008), pp. 8885-96, ISSN 0270-6474

Pandey, S.; Mahato, N. K. & Navale, R. (2010). Role of self-induced sound therapy: Bhramari Pranayama in Tinnitus. *Audiological Medicine,* Vol. 8, No.3, (October 2010), pp. 137-141, ISSN 1651-386X

Patterson, M. B. & Balough, B. J. (2006). Review of Pharmacological Therapy for Tinnitus. *The International Tinnitus Journal,* Vol. 12, No. 2, (June 2006). pp. 149–160, ISSN 0946-5448

Pedemonte, M.; Drexler, D.; Rodio, S.; Geisinger, D.; Bianco, A.; Pol-Fernandes, D. & Bernhardt, V. (2010). Tinnitus treatment with sound stimulation during sleep. *International Tinnitus Journal,* Vol.16, No.1, (March, 2010), pp. 37-43, ISSN 0946-5448

Podoshin, L.; Ben-David, Y.; Fradis, M.; Malatskey, S. & Hafner, H. (1995). Idiopathic subjective tinnitus treated by amitriptyline Hydrochloride/biofeedback. *International Tinnitus Journal,* Vol.1, No.1, (January, 1995), pp. 54-60, ISSN 0946-5448

Ramdev, S. (2005, 2006). *Pranayama: its philosophy and practice,* Divya Prakashan, ISBN 818923501X, Hardwar, India

Rubinstein, J. T. & Tyler, R. S. (2004). Electrical suppression of tinnitus. In: *Tinnitus: Theory and management,* Snow, J.B., pp. 326–335, BC Decker, ISBN 155009243X, Hamilton (ON)

Ruckenstein, M. J.; Hedgepeth, C.; Rafter, K.O.; Montes, M.L. & Bigelow, D.C. (2001). Tinnitus suppression in patients with cochlear implants. *Otology & Neurotology,* Vol.22, No.2, (March 2001), pp. 200–204, ISSN 0030-6665

Saltzman, M. & Ersner, M. S. (1947). A hearing aid for relief of tinnitus aurium. *The Laryngoscope,* Vol.57, No.5, (May 1947), pp. 358–366, ISSN 1531-4995

Samskriti & Franks, J. (1978). *Hatha Yoga: Manual Two,* Himalayan Institute Press, ISBN 089389043X, Pennsylvania

Schlee, W.; Dohrmann, K.; Hartmann, T.; Lorenz, I.; Muller, N.; Elbert, T. & Weisz, N. (2008). Assessment and modification of the tinnitus-related cortical network. *Seminars in Hearing,* Vol.29, No.3, (August 2008), pp. 270-287, ISSN 0734-0451

Searchfield, G. D.; Cameron, H.; Irving, S. & Kobayashi, K. (2010). Sound therapies and instrumentation for tinnitus management. *The New Zealand Medical Journal,* Vol.123, No.1311, (March 2010), pp. 113-167, ISSN 1175 8716

Seidman, M. D. & Babu, S. (2003). Alternative medications and other treatments for tinnitus: Facts from fiction. *Otolaryngologic Clinics of North America,* Vol.36, No.2, (April 2003), pp.359–381, ISSN 0030-6665

Sherman, S. M. (2001). Tonic and burst firing: dual modes of thalamocortical relay. *Trends in Neurosciences,* Vol.24, No.2, (February 2001), pp.122-6, ISSN 0166-2236

Shulman A.; Aran, J, M.; Tonndorf, J.; Feldmann, H. & Vernon, J. A. (1991). *Tinnitus: Diagnosis/Treatment.* Lea & Febiger, ISBN 0812111214, Philadelphia

Shulman, A. (1997). Medical evaluation. In: *Tinnitus: diagnosis/treatment,* A. Shulman; J. Aran; J. Tonndorf; H. Feldman & J.A. Vernon, (Eds.), 253-292, Singular Publishing Group, ISBN 1565939611, San Diego

Shulman, A.; Strashun, A.M.; Afriyie, M.; Aronson, F.; Abel, W. & Goldstein, B. (1995). SPECT Imaging of brain and tinnitus neurotologic/ neurologic implications. The *International Tinnitus Journal,* Vol.1, No.1, n.d., pp. 13–29, ISSN 0946-5448

Sinopoli, S.; Davis, P. B. & Hanley, P. (2007). Tinnitus: addressing neurological, audiological, and psychological aspects with customized therapy. *Hearing Review.* Vol. 14, No.9, (August 2007), pp. 32-35, ISSN 1074-5734

Smits, M.; Kovacs, S.; De Ridder, D.; Peeters, R. R.; Van-Hecke, P. & Sunaert, S. (2007). Lateralization of functional magnetic resonance imaging (fMRI) activation in the auditory pathway of patients with lateralized tinnitus. *Neuroradiology.* Vol.49, No.8, (August 2007), pp. 669–679, ISSN 0028 3940

Speciale, J. & Stahlbrodt, J.E. (1999). Use of ocular compression to induce vagal stimulation and aid in controlling seizures in seven dogs. *Journal of the American Veterinary Medical Association,* Vol.214, No. 5, (March 1999), pp. 663 –665, ISSN 0003-1488

Staller, S. J. (1998). Suppression of tinnitus with electrical stimulation. In: *Tinnitus: Treatment and relief,* J. A. Vernon, 77–90, Allyn & Bacon, ISBN 0-205-05929-5, Needham Heights, Massachusetts

Surr, R. K.; Montgomery, A. A. & Mueller, H. G. (1985). Effect of amplification on tinnitus among new hearing aid users. *Ear and Hearing,* Vol.6, No.2, (April 1985), pp. 71–75, ISSN 0196-0202

Swadlow, H.A. & Gusev, A. G. (2001). The impact of 'bursting' thalamic impulses at a neocortical synapse. *Nature Neuroscience,* Vol.4, No.4, (April 2001), pp.402-408, ISSN 1097-6256

Sweetow, R. W. & Sabes, J. H. (2010). Effects of acoustical stimuli delivered through hearing aids on tinnitus. *Journal of the American Academy of Audiology,* Vol.21, No.7, (August 2010), pp. 461-473, ISSN 1050-0545

Sweetow, R. W. (2000). Cognitive-behavior modification. In: *Tinnitus handbook,* R. Tyler, (Ed.), 297–311, Singular Publishing Group, ISBN 1-56593-922-0, San Diego (CA)

Sweetow, R. W., & Henderson, S. J. (2010): An overview of common procedures for the management of tinnitus patients. *Hearing Journal,* Vol. 63, No.11, (November 2010), pp. 11-12, 14-15, ISSN 0745-7472

Tyler, R. (2006). *Tinnitus Treatment: Clinical Protocols,* Thieme, ISBN 1-58890-181-5, New York

Tyler, R. S. (1995). Tinnitus in the profoundly hearing-impaired and the effects of cochlear implants. *The Annals of otology, rhinology & laryngology Supplement,* Vol.165, (April 1995), pp. 25–30, ISSN 0096-8056

Tyler, R.S. & Bentler, R.A. (1987). Tinnitus maskers and hearing aids for tinnitus. Seminars in Hearing, Vol.8, No.1, pp. 49-61, ISSN 0734-0451

Tyler, R.S.; Coelho, C. & Noble, W. (2006). Tinnitus: standard of care, personality differences, genetic factors. *Journal for oto-rhino-laryngology and its related specialties,* Vol.68, No.1, (March, 2006), pp. 14-19, ISSN 0301-1569

Vernon, J. A. & Meikle, M. B. (2000). Tinnitus Masking, In: *Tinnitus Handbook,* R. Tyler, (Ed.), 313-356, Singular Thomson Learning, ISBN 1-56593-922-0, San Diego, USA

Vernon, J. A. (1977). Attempts to relieve tinnitus. *Journal of the American Audiology Society,* Vol.2, No. 4, (February 1977), pp. 124–131, ISSN 0360-9294

Vernon, J. A. (2000). Masking of tinnitus through a cochlear implant. The *Journal of the American Academy of Audiology,* Vol.11, No.6, (June 2000), pp. 293–94, ISSN 1050-0545

Vialatte, F. B.; Bakardjiian, H.; Prasad. R. & Cichocki, A. (2009). EEG Paroxysmal Gamma waves during Bhramari Pranayama: a yoga breathing technique. *Consciousness and Cognition,* Vol.18, No.4, (December 2009), pp. 977-88, ISSN 1053-8100

Weisz, N.; Moratti, S.; Meinzer, M.; Dohrmann, K. & Elbert, T. (2005). Tinnitus Perception and Distress Is Related to Abnormal Spontaneous Brain Activity as Measured by Magnetoencephalography. *PLoS Medicine,* Vol.2, No.6, (June 2005), pp. e153, ISSN 1549-1676

Weisz, N.; Muller, S.; Schlee, W.; Dohrmann, K.; Hartmann, T. & Elbert, T. (2007). The neural code of auditory phantom perception. *Journal of Neuroscience,* Vol.27, No.6, (February 2007), pp.1479–1484, ISSN 0270-6474

White, T. P.; Hoffman, S.R. & Gale, E. N. (1986). Psychophysiological therapy for tinnitus, *Ear and Hearing,* Vol.7, No.6, (December, 1986), pp. 397-399, ISSN 0196-0202

Wilson, P. H.; Henry, J.L.; Andersson, G.; Hallman, R.S. & Lindberg, P. (1998). A critical analysis of directive counseling as a component of tinnitus retraining therapy. *British Journal of Audiology,* Vol.32, No.5, (October 1998), pp. 273-286, ISSN 0300-5364

Zabara, J. (1992). Inhibition of experimental seizures in canines by repetitive vagal nerve stimulation. *Epilepsia,* Vol.33, No.6, (November, 1992), pp. 1005 - 1012, ISSN 0013-9580

Zachriat, C. & Kroner-Herwig, B. (2004). Treating chronic tinnitus: comparison of cognitive behavioural and habituation-based treatments. *Cognitive Behaviour Therapy,* Vol.33, No.4, (November, 2010), pp.187-198, ISSN 1650-6073

Part 8

Emotional Side of Tinnitus

10

The "Emotional Side" of Subjective Tinnitus

Roberto Teggi[1], Daniela Caldirola[2], Giampaolo Perna[2,3] and Mario Bussi[1]
[1]*Department of Otolaryngology, Vita-Salute University, San Raffaele Hospital, Milan,*
[2]*Department of Clinical Neuroscience, San Benedetto Hospital, Hermanas Hospitalarias, Albese con Cassano,*
[3]*Department of Psychiatry and Neuropsychology, Faculty of Health, Medicine and Life Sciences, University of Maastricht, Maastricht,*
[1,2]*Italy*
[3]*The Netherlands*

1. Introduction

Tinnitus has been defined as the perception of a sound which cannot be attributed to an external source. Objective tinnitus refers to a rare number of patients in whom sound can be audible to others; for example, a pulsatile sound may be generated by a blood vessel adjacent to the middle ear, or tinnitus may be provoked by a palatal myoclonus. On the other hand, the term "subjective tinnitus" refers to the most common form, in which the source cannot be identified. It is a relatively common symptom and the prevalence is estimated at between 6% and 30% of the total population (Quaranta et al., 1996; Leske et al., 1991).

The underlying physiological mechanisms are largely unknown. A "hearing damage", possibly recovered, is thought to be the causal event. Some authors have pointed out that, after cochlear damage, a cascade of changes occurs in the central auditory pathways and some of these may serve as "neural code" for tinnitus (Eggermont & Roberts, 2004).

Recent papers have demonstrated changes in patients having tinnitus with enhanced spontaneous firing rates in central acoustic pathways (Kaltenbach et al., 2005) and tonotopic reorganization of the auditory cortex with altered synchronous cortical activity (Seki & Eggermont, 2003; Weisz et al., 2007). As a possible demonstration of this theory, repetitive Transcranial Magnetic Stimulation has been demonstrated to be useful in tinnitus treatment (De Ridder et al., 2011).

In clinical practice, the pitch and loudness of tinnitus can be assessed using "psychoacoustic measures"; moreover, in some patients, tinnitus may disappear for a short period after exposure to other sounds (Tyler, 2000).

However, according to the theory of Jastreboff, the tinnitus signal does not always extend beyond the auditory system and in these patients, tinnitus can be perceived only when the subject focuses on it; chronic and disabling tinnitus, on the other hand, is related to inappropriate activation of the limbic system. It has been stated that "perception and reaction to tinnitus are not the same thing" (Hallam et al., 1988).

2. Neurological correlates of tinnitus

2.1 The acoustic pathways

According to most authors, cochlear damage is supposed to be the initiating factor of tinnitus, leading to altered patterns of neural activity along the central auditory pathways. Studies on both animals and humans have been carried out in recent years to assess central areas involved in tinnitus perception. The pathophysiology of tinnitus may be compared with phantom pain felt in subjects with amputated limbs; in both cases, the brain continues to convey perceptual experiences even after the loss of function of peripheral sensory cells (Rauschenecker, 1999). Thus, tinnitus is thought to originate from plastic reorganization (remapping) of auditory pathways and the cortex.

Studies on both animals and humans have been carried out to demonstrate this theory.

In mammals, after a noise or drug-induced hearing loss, an increased spontaneous neural firing rate has been reported in the inferior colliculus, medial geniculate body and auditory cortex (Salvi et al., 2000). It may be of some interest to emphasize that, within the inferior colliculus, spontaneous activity changes are most prominent in neurons tuned to the frequencies of hearing loss, most frequently high frequencies (Chen & Jastreboff, 1995); moreover, in the primary auditory cortex, a drug-induced hearing loss provoked an increased spontaneous firing rate in neurons tuned to high pitched sounds and a decreased firing rate has been demonstrated in neurons tuned to low frequencies (Eggermont & Komiya, 2000). As a result of this remapping, frequency regions adjacent to the deafferented area "invade" the vacated space and become overrepresented in the cortical area.

Not unlike animals, recent studies with EEG, magnetoencephalography (MEG), high resolution MRI and fMRI on humans have demonstrated that tinnitus is associated with changes in cortical and subcortical brain activity (Muhlnickel et al., 2003). Studies with MEG in humans with tinnitus demonstrated a shift of the auditory cortical frequency map at the position of tinnitus frequency, and the entity of the finding was correlated with the strength of tinnitus. Moreover, tinnitus is not only related to reorganization of the omolateral auditory cortex but also to increased gamma-band activity in the controlateral auditory cortex; the entity of this reorganization showed a positive correlation with the severity of tinnitus (Van der Loo, 2009). Further MEG data indicated the possibility that tinnitus may be linked to abnormal spontaneous gamma band activity generated as a consequence of a cochlear disorder in thalamic nuclei, particularly in the medial geniculate body. According to this model, in these deafferented regions, oscillatory alpha activity decreases to theta band activity; as a result, lateral inhibition is reduced, inducing a surrounding gamma band activity, which is known as "the edge effect" (Llinas et al., 2005).

It should be concluded that tinnitus arises from a long-term reorganization of the auditory pathways, particularly at the thalamic and cortical level. Nonetheless, tinnitus has been reported to occur in individuals with normal hearing. "Normal hearing" is determined with pure tone audiometry only at frequencies below 8 kHz; when testing is performed at finer intervals (half octave) and on frequencies above 8 kHz, cases of individuals with tinnitus without hearing loss become rarer (Salvi et al., 2009).

It may be stated that the great majority of tinnitus cases involve hearing loss, although not permanent; nonetheless, the reverse is not true, since not everyone with a permanent sensorineural hearing loss develops tinnitus.

2.2 The role of the limbic system

Patients with chronic tinnitus often present anxiety and depressive disorders, indicating the possibility of an involvement of brain areas related to emotions. Moreover, the loudness of tinnitus seldom correlates with the distress.

In a Voxel Based Morphometry (VBM) study, Muhlau et al. (2006) demonstrated a significant volume loss in the subcallosal area of tinnitus sufferers; results have been replicated in other works, and other limbic structures have been found to be involved in the phenomenon (Landgrebe et al., 2009; Vanneste et al., 2010).

According to the authors, the volume loss may be implicated in characteristic functional consequences. The subcallosal area is a poorly delineated area of the brain and constitutes a major hub linking limbic affective areas and the thalamo-cortical system involved in perception.

Activation of the subcallosal area, for example, correlates with the unpleasant effects of dissonant music (Blood et al., 1999); patients with depressive disorders often present abnormal activity levels in this area (Mayberg et al., 2005). Moreover, the subcallosal area overlaps with the Nucleus Accumbens (NA), the major component of the ventral striatum (Gruber et al., 2009). The NA contains both dopaminergic and serotoninergic fibres. The dopaminergic system has been demonstrated to play an important role in reward behaviour and avoidance learning (McCullogh et al., 1993), while serotoninergic fibres modulate emotional responses to external stimuli. Finally, the NA receives glutamatergic fibres from the Amygdala, Hippocampus and Raphe Nuclei, and the latter are responsible for the regulation of sleep (Ambroggi et al., 2008).

Anatomical studies have tried to demonstrate the connections between the Thalamic Reticular Nucleus (TRN), Medial Geniculate Nucleus (MGN) and the limbic system. The thalamic system without doubt plays an important role in transmission of sensorial information to cortical areas.

It has recently been demonstrated that TRN GABAergic afferent fibres strongly inhibit the neural activity of the MGN in animals, and its activity is highly frequency-specific (Yu et al., 2009). On the other hand, the TRN receives serotoninergic afferents from the limbic system (particularly the Dorsal Raphe, NA) with excitatory function on TRN neurons (McCormick & Wang, 1991). The network has been defined as "the noise cancellation system" (Rauschecker, 2010).

According to Rauschecker (2010), the maintenance of tinnitus may be linked to two possibilities:

It may be a consequence of overload from chronic firing of limbic system neurons, trying to compensate for the tinnitus signal.

It is possible that tinnitus patients have an independent, systemic vulnerability in one or more limbic transmitter system, particularly serotonin, making these individuals more susceptible to tinnitus as well as other disorders such as chronic pain or depression; in these subjects, the level of transmitters may decline more rapidly than in unaffected persons.

The first possibility is in accordance with previous theories which assigned a central role to auditory dysfunction and a reactive role to the limbic system. The second possibility underlines a possible more central role of the limbic system in preventing perception and chronicization of tinnitus.

3. The "emotional side" of tinnitus

Many studies have focused on the emotional aspect of tinnitus. Tinnitus has been demonstrated to be an important stressor and is often associated with anxiety and, in particular, depression.

Individuals unable to eliminate tinnitus with medical therapies may perceive the problem as permanent; if the tinnitus persists, patients tend to exhaust their coping resources and experience negative emotions. Similarities have been found with the experience of living with chronic pain, since both disorders are intractable, subjective and unpleasant and both significantly modify the life of sufferers.

Several studies have focused on the link between tinnitus and emotional distress. The onset of tinnitus often constitutes a change in a person's life and leads to significant psychological disturbance. According to McKenna et al. (1991), 45% of patients with tinnitus were in need of psychological help, and 86% of these subjects accepted it. Moreover, the onset of tinnitus is often associated with stress, and tinnitus annoyance may increase during stressful periods (Schmitt et al., 2000). Other stresses may aggravate tinnitus annoyance; in a sample of air traffic controllers suffering from tinnitus, a period of workload contributed to an increased perception of tinnitus. Moreover, other health problems can have additive effects as stressors and increase the probability of developing disability, social isolation and low levels of enjoyment of life (Vogt & Kastner, 2002). Anyway, the relationship between stress and tinnitus is still under debate; if tinnitus can be exacerbated by stress and fatigue, some stress-tolerant people might tolerate higher degrees of tinnitus and even when stress increases, subjective tinnitus does not (Hebert & Lupien, 2009).

3.1 Tinnitus, anxiety and depressive disorders

Without doubt, there is an association between tinnitus annoyance and a poor psychological state. Anxiety and depression play an important role in the tinnitus process and often the characteristics of tinnitus do not predict the distress provoked by it.

The relationship between tinnitus distress and psychological disorders has been widely investigated. Sullivan et al. (1988) studied the association between disabling tinnitus and affective disorders. Tinnitus sufferers presented a greater lifetime prevalence of major depression and current major depression than a control group of subjects with hearing loss without tinnitus. Moreover, patients with tinnitus and depressive disorders presented a higher psychosocial disability than non-depressive tinnitus sufferers, while no difference was established between patients with tinnitus without depression and controls with hearing loss. The authors concluded that the results are in accordance with the hypothesis that disability is strongly associated with depression.

Scott & Lindberg (2000) studied the psychological profiles and somatic complaints in two groups of tinnitus sufferers, respectively, help-seeking and non-help-seeking for tinnitus. They tried to address the question whether the two groups presented differences in psychological and somatic profiles. The groups differed both on the trait and state scales for anxiety, depression and reaction to stress even when hearing impairment was controlled. Help-seeking patients also showed a pattern of increased vulnerability. The authors concluded that the link between anxiety, depression, reactions to stress and chronic tinnitus is confirmed. Subjects with disabling tinnitus are more burdened with more severe somatization problems which might result in a less adaptive repertoire of coping strategies.

Results somehow confirm the data in an earlier paper (Halford & Anderson, 1991) in which the authors found that tinnitus was associated with a high anxiety trait and depression. The severity of tinnitus was correlated with both anxiety and depression but coefficients were of low magnitude. As a result, it may be argued that more anxious subjects with a negative outlook more probably will be unable to realize helpful coping strategies; anxiety and depression may predispose subjects to pay greater attention to tinnitus and related negative effects. Significantly, Andersson (1996) found that the predisposition toward optimism assessed by the Life Orientation Scale was negatively correlated with tinnitus complaints.

3.2 Coping style

Coping has been defined as the efforts to reduce the negative impacts of stress on individual well-being. Coping efforts are triggered by the appraisal of situations or symptoms as threatening, harmful or anxiety producing.

Studies concerning coping strategies in patients with tinnitus arise from the practical consideration that tinnitus is a relatively common symptom and it only becomes a disabling problem in a small number of subjects. That is to say, most sufferers adjust to tinnitus on their own and this adjustment does not appear to be closely related to the severity of the condition.

Budd & Pugh (1996), in their exhaustive work, assessed coping strategies using the 40-item Tinnitus Coping Style Questionnaire (TCSQ). They identified two different coping styles. The first one, termed "maladaptative", was characterized by the failure to avoid tinnitus. Sufferers reported that they often dream about life without tinnitus and pray that their tinnitus would go away. The coping style was characterized by catastrophic thinking about the consequences of tinnitus and these patients worry that tinnitus may cause a nervous breakdown. These subjects are often unable to cope with the noises and they attempt to get away from tinnitus by avoiding social situations. This coping style was associated with increased levels of tinnitus severity, anxiety and depression.

The second coping strategy was defined as "effective coping" and was characterized by sufferers' acceptance of tinnitus and using a broad range of adaptive coping strategies including positive self-talk, distraction and attention switching. These patients often reported increasing daily activities and taking up new hobbies and interests. According to the authors, this coping style was not correlated with decreased tinnitus severity; nonetheless, this coping style was not correlated with anxiety and depression.

3.3 Impact of tinnitus on life

It may be said that, in some cases, tinnitus has a considerable impact on work, sleep, family relationships and, more generally, on way of life.

Several studies have investigated the effects of tinnitus on people's ability to work. Surprisingly, in only a few cases did tinnitus sufferers refer to having difficulties in their jobs and only a few subjects were unable to work. Above all, people performing jobs requiring precision or working with music (music performers, sound technicians) were most disabled in their working life (Andersson, 2000a; Vallianatou et al., 2001).

On the other hand, sleep is without doubt the most important problem in everyday life for patients with tinnitus. Questionnaire-based studies (Sanchez & Stephens, 1997) concluded that sleep disturbance is probably the most common problem, since 71% of patients reported it. Davis et al. (1995) found that, in a normal population sample, 5% had sleep disorders and tinnitus was the causal factor.

Since patients with tinnitus often display a range of behaviours to communicate their distress to other people, marital support may play a significant role in coping style. In a questionnaire-based study on 91 tinnitus sufferers and 74 spouses, Pugh et al. (2004) reported that solicitous responses, that is to say, sympathetic responses to complaints about tinnitus, were directly and positively related to a maladaptive coping style; on the other hand, punitive responses were directly and positively related to anxiety and depression, both of which in turn mediated a relationship between punishing and maladaptive coping and tinnitus severity. Overlapping results have been found by Sullivan et al. (2004). Both papers underlined the role of familiar relationships in coping styles and the central role of depression in tinnitus distress.

3.4 Tinnitus and cognitive impairment

Tinnitus sufferers often complain of difficulties in cognitive functioning, particularly poor attention and concentration in everyday activities. In a recent paper, Hallam et al. (2004) investigated cognitive tasks with a self-administered questionnaire; the questionnaire measured performance under single and dual task conditions and results were compared with those of a group of patients with hearing impairment and a group of non-clinical subjects. Tinnitus patients responded significantly more slowly than the other groups; in general, comparisons on the other tasks demonstrated equivalent performance, even though tinnitus and hearing loss groups performed more poorly than non-clinical group on verbal fluency. The authors concluded that cognitive inefficiency in tinnitus subjects may be related to the control of attentional processes, similar to published findings on the effects of chronic pain on cognitive processes.

Considering the often present comorbid of hearing loss, this may be a possible bias in the evaluation of cognitive processes in tinnitus sufferers.

Andersson et al. (2000b) assessed the performances of tinnitus patients and healthy controls with normal hearing on three versions of the Stroop test. Patients scored significantly higher than controls on the Beck Depression Inventory(BDI) and the Spielberger Trait State Anxiety Inventory (STAI-S), but these measures did not correlate with the Stroop results. The authors concluded that the results indicate that tinnitus patients have impaired cognitive performance overall, but hearing impairment cannot be excluded as a possible confounder.

As a final consideration, recent papers have demonstrated inefficiencies in cognitive processes in tinnitus patients, but the real "weight" of mood disorders and of more practical problems (i.e. hearing loss) in it is still unclear. Moreover, it seems possible that tinnitus interferes more with mundane tasks than with high priority tasks in everyday life.

3.5 Tinnitus and personality trait

As previously described, the association between tinnitus and psychological state has been widely investigated, but at present, the results are unclear; tinnitus sufferers are often comorbid for anxiety and depression and the more depressed patients experience a higher distress with tinnitus. On the other hand, the association between tinnitus and personality trait is still under debate. That is to say, will tinnitus provoke distress, particularly in predisposed subjects, with a peculiar personality profile? After all, Jastreboff & Hazel (1993) found no differences in psychoacoustic measures of tinnitus (intensity, frequency and minimum suppression level) among patients with high and low annoyance.

Meric et al. (1998) and Vallianatou et al. (2001), found no peculiar personality profile in their subjects with chronic tinnitus assessed with the Minnesota Multiphasic Personality

Inventory (MMPI), even though the first authors found a correlation between MMPI depression scale and the Tinnitus Handicap Questionnaire.

On the other hand, Erlandsson et al. (2000) reported a rate of 50% of personality disorders in tinnitus sufferers, which is significantly higher than the 10-13% that the author estimated in the normal population.

Recent papers have focused on the relationship between tinnitus distress and type D personality. The definition "type D" (D stands for Distressed) has been introduced in psychology to describe a joint personality trait between negative affectivity and social inhibition. Type D personality can be assessed with a 14-item questionnaire, the Type D Scale (DS14).

Negative affectivity (NA) refers to the tendency to experience negative emotions across time/situations. High-NA individuals experience more feelings of dysphoria, anxiety, and irritability, have a negative view of self and scan the world for signs of impending trouble.

Social Inhibition (SI) refers to the tendency to inhibit the expression of emotions/behaviours in social interactions to avoid disapproval by others. High-SI individuals tend to feel inhibited, tense, and insecure when with others. Individuals with type D personality show a high vulnerability to chronic distress. Finally, Type D patients are at risk for clustering of psychological risk factors, including depression, anxiety, and irritability, and low levels of self-esteem, well-being, and positive affect.

Type D personality has been associated with post-traumatic stress disorders, hypertension, sudden cardiac arrest, development of cancer, and more widely with all-cause mortality (Denollet, 2005).

Bartels et al. (2010) studied personality trait in 265 patients with chronic tinnitus and the results were compared with a group of ENT patients without tinnitus. Patients demonstrated a higher level of neuroticism, negative affectivity and social inhibition and a lower level of extraversion and emotional stability than controls. According to the authors, the type D personality is independently associated with tinnitus and the prediction of developing chronic tinnitus is improved with the addition of type D personality to the single personality traits.

3.6 Therapies for tinnitus and psychiatric disorders

Over the last decade, repetitive Transcranial Magnetic Stimulation (rTMS) has received increasing attention as a potential therapeutic tool for tinnitus. Therapy is based on the application of a magnetic field on the scalp, inducing an electrical modification in specific areas of the brain. It has been demonstrated that rTMS directly modulates electrical activity in superficial areas of the brain but induces indirect modifications in remote areas which are connected to the stimulated zone. Low frequency rTMS on the left temporo-parietal cortex has been demonstrated to be useful in the treatment of tinnitus, nonetheless, some doubts arise about maintenance of therapeutic results (Langguth et al., 2008).

Recently, encouraging results have been obtained with the application of low frequency rTMS on prefrontal areas (Vanneste et al., 2011); the authors reported a significant reduction in both tinnitus intensity and distress. They hypothesized that results may be linked to modulation of the Anterior Cingulate Cortex (ACC), which plays an important role in the integration of motivationally important information with bodily responses related to the survival of individuals. The authors propose that a possible function of the ACC in tinnitus could be related to the fact that the generated phantom sound is considered as motivationally important and the ACC responds with the maintenance of tinnitus in the focus of attention.

It may be of some importance that prefrontal cortex rTMS has been demonstrated to be useful in the therapy of psychiatric diseases including depression, panic and posttraumatic stress disorders (George et al., 2009).

A review of drug therapy for tinnitus is beyond the goals of this chapter; nonetheless, it must be underlined that among antidepressants, Selective Serotonin Reuptake Inhibitors (SSRIs) have been demonstrated to have probably the best efficacy in the treatment of tinnitus distress (Folmer & Shi, 2004).

4. Preliminary data from our research study on patients with chronic tinnitus. The role of psychological and clinical variables in tinnitus-related handicap and distress

As previously described, peculiar personality profiles, such as type D personality, pessimism and impulsiveness traits, inefficient coping abilities and anxiety and depressive symptoms have been associated with high intrusiveness of tinnitus and high tinnitus-related distress. Several personality profiles and cognitive constructs have been implicated in other medically unexplained somatic symptoms or in medical condition-related distress (Russo et al., 1994) and may also be involved in modulating the impact of tinnitus on quality of life. Thus, in a sample of patients with chronic tinnitus, we investigated the relationship between tinnitus-related distress and temperamental and character dimensions, according to Cloninger's theory of personality (Cloninger et al., 1993), cognitive constructs of worry and fear associated with common physical sensations. Moreover, we investigated the role of anxiety and depressive symptoms in mediating the influence of personality dimensions and cognitive constructs on the impact of tinnitus in everyday life.

4.1 Subjects

Forty-eight subjects suffering from unilateral tinnitus were recruited, out of those participating in an randomized double-blind study performed to assess the efficacy of low-level laser treatment for tinnitus (Teggi et al., 2009) and who also agreed to take part in this section of the study. They were all outpatients at the ENT Department of San Raffaele Hospital, Milan, Italy. Twenty-five were males and 23 were females and their mean age was 52.2 ± 11.9 years; the mean duration of illness was 61.2 ± 72.7 months. They all had sensorineural hearing loss, stable during the previous 3 months, from causes such as presbycusis, Ménière's disease, or idiopathic sudden sensorineural hearing loss. The day the patients received the laser treatment devices and instructions, they were further assessed with a self-administered battery of psychological tests; detailed explanations for test compilation were provided by expert psychologists.

4.2 Clinical and psychological measures

All subjects underwent pure tone audiometry and a complete psychoacoustic assessment, including pitch, loudness, minimum masking level and loudness discomfort level. In this section of the study, we focused on loudness and minimum masking level (MML) as the main measures of tinnitus intensity experienced by the subjects. Loudness match was determined by balancing the loudness of the tinnitus with the loudness of a tone at pitch

frequency in the contralateral ear and was expressed in decibel sensation level. The minimum masking level was established using broadband noise; first, the monaural hearing threshold was obtained, and then raised until the patient reported that the tinnitus was inaudible. Both loudness and minimum masking level were determined using 1-dB steps.
Tinnitus distress was assessed with the Tinnitus Handicap Inventory (THI) (Newman et al., 1996). This is a 25-item self-administered questionnaire for the measurement of tinnitus handicap and the impact of tinnitus on everyday functioning (total score ranging from 0 to 100, with a higher score indicating greater handicap). Depression and anxiety levels were assessed with the 31-item Self-Evaluation Depression Scale (SAD) and the 20-item State-Trait Anxiety Inventory, State Form (STAI-Y-1), respectively. Different psychological constructs were assessed with the following self-rating tests: the 17-item Body Sensation Questionnaire (BSQ), measuring fear associated with common physical sensations, such as heart palpitations, dizziness, nausea; the 16-item Penn State Worry Questionnaire (PSWQ), assessing the trait dimension of the worry process and its excessiveness, duration and uncontrollability, regardless of the contents of worry; the 5-item Physical Treat domain of the Worry Domains Questionnaire (WDQ), assessing worry specifically with regard to health-related content; the 240-item Temperament and Character Inventory-Revised (TCI-R), assessing the four temperamental dimensions (Novelty Seeking, NS; Harm Avoidance, HA; Reward Dependence, RD; Persistence, P) and three character dimensions (Self-Directedness, SD; Cooperativeness, C; Self-Transcendence, ST) of the 7-factor psychobiological model of personality proposed by Cloninger et al. (1993).

4.3 Statistical analyses and results

Pearson zero-order and partial correlation were performed to evaluate the association between the psychological constructs and the level of tinnitus-related distress as measured by the THI. Zero-order correlation measures the raw observed linear association between two variables, while partial correlation allows us to study the degree of association between two variables removing the effect of a set of controlling variables. Preliminary analyses were performed to evaluate whether sociodemographic (gender, age, years of education), duration of illness, psychoacoustic variables (loudness, MML), level of anxiety (STAI-Y-1, mean value) and level of depression (SAD) were significantly associated with the psychological variables considered (BSQ, WDQ-PT, PSWQ, TCI-R) or with THI. Zero-order correlation was performed to evaluate the association among continuous variables while an independent sample *t*-test was performed for the association between a continuous and a dichotomous variable (gender). If significant associations were found, these variables were inserted as controlling variables in the partial correlation analyses evaluating the association between psychological constructs and level of tinnitus-related distress.
Preliminary analyses showed that age, gender and years of education (mean value 11.7±13.8 years) did not significantly correlate with any psychological dimensions or with THI scores (mean value 45.3± 28.0). Similarly, neither duration of illness nor loudness (mean value 6.7±5.5) and MML (mean value 8.7±5.7) were significantly correlated with THI or with any of the psychological constructs evaluated. On the other hand, anxiety level (STAI-Y-1, mean value 44.6±12.2) and depression level (SAD, mean value 49.08±12.07) were significantly correlated with several of the psychological dimensions considered. Furthermore, they were strongly correlated with tinnitus-related distress as measured by THI scores. Thus, we inserted anxiety and depression levels as controlling variables in the partial correlation

analyses, whereas we excluded sociodemographic and psychoacoustic variables due to the lack of association found in preliminary analyses.
Correlations between tinnitus-related distress and psychological variables revealed THI to be significantly and positively related to the Penn State Worry Questionnaire scores, the Physical Treat domain of the Worry Domains Questionnaire scores and the Harm Avoidance temperamental dimension, whereas it was negatively related to the Self-Directedness and Cooperativeness character dimensions. When SAD was inserted as controlling variable, no partial correlations between THI and the considered psychological constructs remained significant. With the insertion of STAI-Y-1 as controlling variable, only the partial correlations between THI and the Penn State Worry Questionnaire scores and between THI and the Physical Treat domain of the Worry Domains Questionnaire scores remained significant, whereas all of the other correlations were not significant.

4.4 Conclusions

Our results showed that the levels of handicap and distress related to tinnitus were not related either to the psychoacoustic measures of tinnitus (perceived loudness or minimum masking level) or to the duration of illness or individual variables such as age, gender, or year of education. On the other hand, patients with high levels of tinnitus-related distress showed a temperamental and character profile with high Harm Avoidance temperamental dimension (i.e. subjects characterized by pessimism, anticipatory anxiety and fear of uncertainty, shyness, insecurity of the unknown, fatigue and lack of energy) and low Self-Directedness (i.e. subjects characterized by immaturity, poor accountability, weak capacity to focus on personal objectives) and Cooperativeness (i.e. subjects characterized by a tendency to isolation, lack of empathy, poor ability to collaborate with others) character dimensions. Similarly, the cognitive profile with high proneness to worry, including worry on health-related content, and high sensitivity and fear towards somatic sensations, was associated with high THI scores. Finally, high tinnitus-related distress was related to severity of anxiety and depressive symptoms. However, the impact of personality and cognitive profiles on tinnitus-related distress appeared to be strongly influenced by anxiety and depressive symptoms; indeed, only the proneness to worry seemed to have a direct association with high THI scores even when anxiety levels were taken into account.
Overall, our results support the idea that individual differences in personality and cognitive profiles may play a relevant role in modulating the impact of tinnitus on the quality of life, over and above the perceived loudness of the tinnitus itself, but underscore the importance of anxiety and depressive symptoms in mediating this association. Thus, in clinical settings, the specific assessment of severity of anxiety and depressive symptoms in patients with tinnitus and high THI scores is highly recommended; specific treatments directed toward the reduction of these symptoms may be an important therapeutic resource and may, in turn, improve the efficacy of psychological treatments focusing on the personality and cognitive traits that worsen the impact of tinnitus on the quality of life.
As a final consideration, the previous approach to the problem of the relationship between tinnitus and psychiatric disorders was univocal; tinnitus may provoke in some individual a strong emotional response. Recent studies focused on the possibility that annoyance, which is the "real problem", is the result of the action of tinnitus on subjects with a predisposing personality trait. Moreover, future goal should be to assess the role of serotoninergic system in the maintenance and distress provoked by tinnitus. Since SSRIs demonstrated to be useful

in the treatment of tinnitus, it may be hypothesized that the action is strictly related to its activity on "mood system" in the brain or a direct action on acoustic pathways may be supposed (the "noise cancellation system").

5. References

Ambroggi, F.; Ishikawa, A.; Fields, H.L.; Nicola, SM. (2008) Basolateral amygdala neurons facilitate renard seeking behavior by exciting nucleus accumbens neurons. *Neuron*, Vol. 59, Issue 4, pp. 648-61, ISSN 0896-6273.

Andersson G. (1996) The role of optimism in patients with tinnitus and in patients with hearing impairment. *Psychol Health*, Vol. 11, Issue 5, pp. 697-707, ISSN 0887-0446.

Andersson G. (2000a) Longitudinal follow-up of occupational status in tinnitus patients. *Int Tinnitus J*, Vol. 6, Issue 2, Issue, pp. 127-9, ISSN 0946-5448.

Andersson, G.; Eriksson, J.; Lundth, L.G.; Lyttkens, L. (2000b) Tinnitus and cognitive interference: a Stroop paradigm study. *J Speech Lang Her Res*, Vol. 43, Issue 5, pp. 1168-73, ISSN 1092-4388.

Bartels, H.; Middel, B.; Pedersen, S.S.; Staal, M.J.; Albers, F.W.J. (2010) The distressed (Type D) personality is independently associated with tinnitus: a case-control study. *Psychosomatics*, Vol. 51, Issue 1, pp. 29-38, ISSN 0033-3182.

Blood, AJ.; Zatorre, RJ.; Bermudez, P.; Evans, AC. (1999) Emotional responses to pleasant and unpleasant music correlate with activity in paralimbic brain regions. *Nat Neurosci*, Vol. 2, Issue 4, pp. 382-7, ISSN 1097-6256.

Budd, RJ; Pugh R. (1996). Tinnitus coping style and its relationship to tinnitus severity and emotional distress. *J Psychosom Res*, Vol. 41, Issue 4, pp. 327-35, ISSN 0022-3999.

Chen, G. & Jastreboff, P.J. (1995) Salycilate induced abnormal activity in the inferior colliculus of rats. *Hear Res.*, Vol 82, Issue 2, pp. 158-78, ISSN 0378-5955.

Cloninger, C.L.; Svrakic, D.M.; Przybeck, T.R. (1993) A psychobiological model of temperament and character. *Arch Gen Psychiatry*, Vol 50, Issue 12, pp. 975-90, ISSN 0003-990X.

Davis, A. (1995) *Hearing in adults*. Whurr Publisher, ISBN 1861564031 London.

Denollet J. (2000) DS14: standard assessment of negative affectivity, social inhibition, and Type D personality. *Psychosom Me*, Vol. 67 Issue 1, pp.89-97, ISSN 0033-3174.

De Ridder, D; Vanneste, S; Kovacs, S; Sunaert, S; Menovsky, T; Van de Heyning, P; Moller, A. (2011) Transcranial Magnetic stimulation and extradural electrodes. implanted on secondary auditory cortex for tinnitus suppression *J Neurosurg*. [epub ahead of print], ISSN 1933-0693.

Eggermont, J.J. & Komiya H. (2000) Moderate noise trauma in juvenile cats results in profound cortical topographic map changes in adulthood. *Hear Res*, Vol 142 Issue 1-2, pp. 89-101 ISSN 0378-5955.

Eggermont, J.J.; Roberts, L.E. (2004) The neuroscience of tinnitus. *Trends Neurosci*, Vol 27, Issue 11, pp. 676–82, ISSN 0166-2236.

Erlandsson S. (2000) Psychological profile of tinnitus patients. In *Tinnitus Handbook.*, Thomson Learning, pp 25-57, ISBN 156-5939-22-0 San Diego, USA.

Folmer, R.L. & Shi, Y.B. (2004) SSRI use by tinnitus patients: interactions between depression and tinnitus severity. *Ear Nose Throat J*, Vol. 83 Issue 2 pp. 107-8, ISSN 0145-5613.

George, M.S.; Padberg, F.; Schlaepfer, T.E.; O'Reardon, J.P.; Fitzgerald, P.B.; Nahas, Z.H.; Marcolin, M.A. (2009) Controversy: repetitive transcranial magnetic stimulation or transcranial direct current stimulation shows efficacy in treating psychiatric diseases (depression, manis, schizophrenia, obsessive-compulsive disorder, panic, posttraumatic stress disorder). *Brain Stimul*, vol 2, Issue 1, pp.14-21, ISSN 1935-861X..

Gruber, AJ; Hussain, RJ; O'Donnell, P. (2009) The Nucleus Accumbens: a switchboard for goal-directed behaviors. *PloS ONE*, Vol 4, Issue 4 pp e5062, ISSN 0005062.

Halford, J.B.; Anderson, S.D. (1991) Anxiety and depression in tinnitus sufferers. *J Psychosom Res*, Vol 35, Issue 4-5, pp. 383-90, ISSN 0022-3999.

Hallam, R.S.; Jakes, S.C.; Hinchcliffe, R. (1988) Cognitive variables in tinnitus annoyance. *Br J Clin Psychol*, Vol.27, Issue 3, pp. 213-22, ISSN 0144-6657.

Hallam, R.S.; McKenna, L.; Shurlock, L. (2004) Tinnitus impairs cognitive processes. *Int J Audiol*, Vol. 43, Issue 4, pp. 218-26, ISSN 1499-2027.

Hebert, S & Lupien, SJ. (2009) Salivary cortisol levels, subjective stress and tinnitus intensity in tinnitus sufferers during noise exposure in the laboratory. *Int J Hyg Environ Health*, Vol. 212, Issue 1, pp. 37-44, ISSN 1438-4639.

Jastreboff, P.J.; Hazell, J.W.P. (1993) A neurophysiological approach to tinnitus: clinical implications. *Br J Audiol*, Vol. 27, Issue 1, pp. 7-17, ISSN 0300-5364.

Kaltenbach, J.A.; Zhang, J.; Finlayson, P. (2005) Tinnitus as a plastic phenomenon and its possible neural underpinnings in the dorsal cochlear nucleus. *Hear Res*, vol.206, Issue 1-2, pp. 220-6, ISSN 0378-5955.

Landgrebe, M.; Langguth, B.; Rosengarth, K.; Braun, S.; Koch, A.; Kleinjung, T., May A.; de Ridder, D.; Hajak, G. (2009) Structural brain changes in tinnitus: grey matter decrease in auditory and non auditory brain areas. *Neuroimage*, Vol 46, Issue 1, pp. 213-8. ISSN 1053-8119.

Langguth, B.; de Ridder, D.; Dornhoffer, J.L.; Eichhammer, P.; Folmer, R.L.; Frank, E.; Fregni, L. et al. (2008) Controversy: Does repetitive transcranial magnetic stimulation/transcranial direct current stimulation show efficacy in treating tinnitus patients? *Brain Stimul*, Vol. 1, Issue 3, pp. 192-205, ISSN 1935-861X.

Leske, M.C. (1981) Prevalence estimates of communicative disorders in the US. Language, hearing and vestibular disorders. *American Speech and Hearing Association*, Vol. 23, Issue 3, pp. 229-37, ISSN 0001-2475.

Llinas, R.R.; Urbano, F.J.; Leznick, E.; Ramirez, R.R.; van Marle, H.J. (2005) Rhythmic and dysrhytmic talamocortical dynamics: GABA system and the edge effect. *Trends Neurosci*, Vol.28, Issue 6, pp. 325-33, ISSN 0166-2236.

Mayberg, H.S.; Lozano A.M.; Voon V.; McNeely H.E.; Seminowicz, D.; Hamani, C.; Schwalb, J.M.; Kennedy, S.H. (2005). Deep brain stimulation for treatment-resistant depression. *Neuron*, Vol. 45, Issue 5, pp. 651-60, ISSN 0896-6273.

Meric, C.; Gartner, M.; Collet, L.; Chery-Croze, S. (1998) Psychopathological profile of tinnitus sufferers: evidence concerning the relationship between tinnitus features and impact on life. *Audiol Neurotol*, Vol 3, Issue 4, pp. 240-52, ISSN 1420-3030.

McCormick, D.A. &Wang Z. (1991) Serotonin and noradrenaline excite GABAergic neurons of the guinea-pig and cat nucleus reticularis thalami. *J Physiol*, Vol. 442 Issue 10, pp. 235-55, ISSN 0022-3751.

McCullough, L.D.; Sokolowski, J.D.; Salamone, J.D. (1993). A neurochemical and behavioural investigation of the involvement of nucleus accumbensdopamine in instrumental avoidance. *Neuroscience*, Vol. 52, Issue 4, pp. 919-25, ISSN 0306-4522.

McKenna, L.; Hallam, R.S.; Hinchcliffe, R. (1991) The prevalence of psychological disturbance in neurotology outpatients. *Clin Otolaryngol Allied Sc,* Vol. 16, Issue 5, pp. 452-6, ISSN 0307-7772.

Muhlau, M.; Rauschecker, J.P.; Oestricher, E.; Gaser, C.; Rottinger, M.; Wohlschlager, A.M.; Simon, F.; Etgen, T.; Conrad, B.; Sanders, D. (2006). Structural brain changes in tinnitus. *Cereb Cortex,* Vol 16, Issue 9, pp. 1283-8, ISSN 1047-3211.

Muhlnickel, W.; Elbert, T.; Taub, E.; Flor, H. (1998) Reorganization of auditory cortex in tinnitus. *Proc Natl Acad Sci USA* Vol. 95, Issue 17, pp. 10340-3, ISSN 0027-8424.

Newman, C.R.; Jacobson, G.P.; Spitzer, J.B. (1996) Development of the Tinnitus Handicap Inventory. Arch Otolaryngol Head Neck Surg, Vol 122, Issue 2, pp. 143-8, ISSN 0886-4470.

Pugh, R.; Stephens, D.; Budd, R. (2004) The contribution of spouse responses and marital satisfaction to the experience of chronic tinnitus. *Audiol Med,* Vol 2, Issue 1, pp. 60-73, ISSN 1651-386X.

Quaranta, A.; Assennato, G.; Sallustio, V. (1996) Epidemiology of hearing problems among adults in Italy. *Scandinavian Audiology,* Vol 42, Suppl. , pp. 7-11, ISSN 0107-8593.

Rauschecker, J.P. (1999) Auditory cortical plasticity: a comparison with other sensory systems. *Trends Neurosci,* Vol. 22, Issue 2, pp. 74-80, ISSN 0166-2236.

Rauschecker, J.P., Leaver, A.M.; Muhlau, M. (2010). Tuning out the noise: limbic-auditory interactions in tinnitus. *Neuron,* Vol. 66, Issue 6, pp. 819-26, ISSN 0896-6273.

Russo, J.; Katon, W.; Sullivan, M.; Clark, M.; Buchwald D. (1994) Severity of somatisation and its relationship to psychiatric disorders and personality. *Psychosomatics,* Vol.35, Issue 6, pp. 546-56, ISSN 0033-3182.

Salvi, R.J.; Wang, J.; Ding D. (2000) Auditory plasticity and hyperactivity following cochlear damage. *Hear Res,* Vol 147, Issue 1-2, pp. 261-74, ISSN 0378-5955.

Salvi, R.J.; Lobarinas, E.; Sun, W. (2009) Pharmacological treatments for tinnitus: new and old. *Drugs Future,* Vol. 34, Issue 5, pp. 381-400, ISSN 0377-8282.

Sanchez, L.; Stephens, D. (1997) A tinnitus problem questionnaire. *Ear Hearing,* Vol 18, Issue 3, pp. 210-7, ISSN 0196-0202.

Seki, S. & Eggermont J.J. (2003) Changes in spontaneous firing rate and neural synchrony in cat primary auditory cortex after localized tone-induced hearing loss. *Hearing Res,* Vol 180, Issue 1-2, pp. 28-38, ISSN 0378-5955.

Schmitt, C., Patak, M.; Kroner-Herwig B. (2000) Stress and the onset of sudden hearing loss and tinnitus. *Tinnitus Journal,* Vol. 6, Issue 1, pp. 41-9, ISSN 0946-5448.

Scott, B.; Lindberg, P. (2000) Psychological profile and somatic complaints between help-seeking and non help-seeking tinnitus subjects. *Psychosomatics,* Vol. 41, Issue 4, pp. 347-52, ISSN 0033-3182.

Sullivan, M.; Katon, W.; Russo, J.; Dobie, R.; Sakai, C. (1994) Coping and marital support as correlates of tinnitus disability *Gen H Psy,* Vol. 16, Issue 4, pp. 259-66, ISSN 0163-8343.

Teggi, R; Bellini, C.; Piccioni, L.O.; Palonta, F.; Bussi M. (2009) Transmeatal low-level laser therapy for chronic tinnitus with coclea dysfunction. *Audiol Neurotol.,* Vol 14, Issue 2, pp. 115-20, ISSN 1420-3030.

Tyler, R.S. (2000) The psychoacoustical measurement of tinnitus. In *Tinnitus Handbook,* Thomson Learning, pp. 149-79, ISBN 156-5939-22-0 San Diego, USA.

Vallianatou, N.; Christodoulu, P.; Nestoros, J.; Helidonis, E. (2001) Audiologic and psychological profile of Greek patients with tinnitus - preliminary findings. *Am J Otolaryngol*, Vol. 22, Issue 2, pp. 33-7, ISSN 0196-0709.

Van der Loo, E.; Gais, S.; Congedo, M.; Vanneste, S.; Plazier, M.; Menovski, T.; et al. (2009) Tinnitus intensity dependent gamma oscillations of the controlateral auditory cortex. *PLoS ONE*, Vol 4, Issue 10, p. e7396, ISSN 1932-6203.

Vanneste S., Plazier M., van der Loo E., de Heyning P.V., Congedo M., De Ridder D. (2010) The neural correlates of tinnitus-related distress. *Neuroimage*, Vol 52, Issue 2, pp.470–480, ISSN 1053-8119.

Vanneste, S.; Plazier, M.; van de Heyning, P.; de Ridder, D. (2011) Repetitive transcranial magnetic stimulation frequency dependent tinnitus improvement by double cone coil prefrontal stimulation. *J Neurol Neurosurg Psychiatry*, Vol [Epub ahead of print], ISSN 0022-3050.

Vogt, J.; Kastner, M. (2002) Tinnituskrankungen be fluglotsen: eine klinisch arbeitpsychologische studie. *Zeitschrift fuer Arbeits und Organisationpsychologie*, Vol. 46, Issue 2, pp. 35-44, ISSN 0007-5868.

Weisz, N.; Muller, S.; Schlee, W.; Dohrmann, K.; Hartmann, T.; Elbert, T. (2007) The neural code of auditory phantom perception. *J Neurosci*, Vol 27, Issue 6, pp. 1479–84, ISSN 0270-6474.

Yu, X.J.; Xu, X.X.; He, S.; He, J. (2009) Change detection by thalamic reticular neurons. *Nat Neurosci*, Vol 12, Issue 9 pp. 1165-70, ISSN 1097-6256.